Dilemmas of Dying
Policies and Procedures for Decisions Not to Treat

Dilemmas of Dying
Policies and Procedures
for Decisions
Not to Treat

Proceedings of a 1979 Conference Sponsored by
Medicine In the Public Interest, Inc.

Edited by

Cynthia B. Wong
Judith P. Swazey

GKH

G. K. Hall Medical Publishers

G. K. Hall Medical Publishers
70 Lincoln Street
Boston, Massachusetts 02111

81 82 83 84 / 4 3 2 1

Dilemmas of dying: policies and procedures for decisions not to treat
    Bibliography.
    1. Right to die—Law and legislation—United States—Congresses. 2. Terminal care—Law and legislation—United States—Congresses. 3. Right to die—Congresses. 4. Terminal care—Moral and religious aspects—Congresses. I. Wong, Cynthia B. II. Swazey, Judith P. III. Medicine In the Public Interest, Inc. IV. Title.
KF3827.E87D54   1979   344'.73'041   79-24943

ISBN 0–8161–2179–6

Contents

Preface

Chartered in 1973, Medicine In the Public Interest, Inc., referred to as MIPI, is a nonprofit corporation involved in studying current issues relating to medicine, science, and society in the United States. In light of the MIPI Board of Directors' long-standing interest in the medical, legal, and ethical issues surrounding the treatment of critically or terminally ill patients, the board decided, in spring 1978, to organize the Dilemmas of Dying Conference. While the Massachusetts Supreme Judicial Court's *Saikewicz* decision was a major impetus for the conference, the issues dealt with transcend the medical-legal particularities of any single state. How decisions are to be made concerning the treatment or nontreatment of critically or terminally ill patients, and by whom, involve questions of values, law, and medicine that need to be addressed not only by health professionals, but also by every segment of society.

Desiring a broad base of professional and public support for the conference, MIPI sought and received the cosponsorship of the Massachusetts Bar Association, the Massachusetts Hospital Association, the Massachusetts Medical Society, the Massachusetts Nurses Association, and WEEI Radio/CBS Boston. MIPI thanks these organizations for their cosponsorship and Eli Lilly Company for the contribution it made toward the preparation of this volume.

The members of the MIPI Board of Directors are also grateful to Dr. Judith P. Swazey, formerly a board member and now the Executive Director, for bringing this important topic to the board's attention, organizing the conference once it was approved, and arranging for publication of this volume. We also thank Mary Claire Adams, MIPI's Administrative Assistant, for arranging and running the conference, Cynthia B. Wong for her outstanding editorial work, and Joan LeVasseur for her patience and persistence in typing the several drafts of these proceedings.

Dana L. Farnsworth, M.D.,
Honorary Chairman, Board
of Directors, Medicine In the
Public Interest, Inc.

Contributors

GEORGE J. ANNAS is Associate Professor of Law and Medicine, Department of Socio-Medical Sciences, Boston University School of Medicine. He received his J.D. from Harvard Law School 1970 and a M.P.H. from the Harvard School of Public Health in 1972, where he was awarded the first Joseph P. Kennedy Foundation Fellowship in Medical Ethics. Among his professional activities, Prof. Annas is Editor-in-Chief of *Medico-Legal News* and Vice-Chairman of the Massachusetts Board of Registration and Discipline in Medicine. His publications include *The Rights of Hospital Patients, Informed Consent to Human Experimentation,* and numerous papers in legal and health care publications.

LOUIS P. BERTONAZZI is a state senator in the Massachusetts Legislature and Adjunct Assistant Professor, Department of Socio-Medical Sciences, Boston University School of Medicine. Sen. Bertonazzi received a B.A. from Tufts University and a M.A. in education from Suffolk University in 1960. Among his many committee and commission assignments in health care and social services, he is Vice-Chairman of the Joint Legislative Committee on Health Care. His honors include the 1978 Annual Division Bronze Medal Award of the American Cancer Society and the 1976 Public Service Award of the Massachusetts Public Health Association.

ROBERT A. BURT is Professor of Law and Co-Chairman of the Program in Law and Medicine at Yale Law School. After earning a B.A. in jurisprudence from Oxford University as a Fulbright Scholar, he received his J.D. from Yale Law School in 1964. In recognition of his work in legal aspects of medicine, Prof. Burt has been elected a fellow of the Institute for Society, Ethics and the Life Sciences and a member of the National Academy of Sciences' Institute of Medicine. His publications include "Authorizing Death for Anomalous Newborns," *Developing Constitutional Rights of, in, and for Children, Standards Relating to Abuse and Neglect,* and *Taking Care of Strangers: The Rule of Law in Doctor-Patient Relations.*

NEIL L. CHAYET is an attorney specializing in health law with the firm of Warner & Stackpole. He received his J.D. from Harvard Law School in 1963. Among his professional activities, Mr. Chayet is a lecturer in legal medicine at Harvard Medical School and a consultant in forensic psychiatry at Massachusetts General Hospital, a member of the Board of Directors, American Society of Law and Medicine, and a legal correspondent for CBS Radio, with a daily presentation on "Looking at the Law." He is the author of *Legal Implications of Emergency Care* and articles and chapters on such medical-legal topics as abortion, drug abuse, mental illness, and informed consent.

HARVEY W. FREISHTAT, a partner in Freishtat and Fried, a law firm specializing in health law, received his J.D. from Harvard Law School in 1972. Mr. Freishtat is a lecturer at The New England School of Law and a member of the Human Studies Committee of the Joslin Diabetes Foundation and the Massachusetts Mental Health Center. He was a major contributor to the volume *Certificate of Need: An Expanding Legislative Concept,* published by Medicine In the Public Interest, Inc., in 1978.

SALLY GADOW is Assistant Professor of Philosophy in the Division of Social Services and Humanities, Department of Community Health and Family Medicine, University of Florida College of Medicine. She received a M.S. in nursing from the University of California, San Francisco, in 1968 and a Ph.D. in philosophy from the University of Texas in 1975. In 1978–1979, she was a fellow in bioethics at the Joseph and Rose Kennedy Institute Center for Bioethics, Georgetown University. Her presentations and publications in health care ethics and the philosophy of medicine include "The Dialectic of Clinical Judgment," "Caring for the Dying: Advocacy or Paternalism?" and *Nursing: Images and Ideals: Opening Dialogue with the Humanities.*

LEONARD H. GLANTZ is Assistant Professor of Law and

Medicine, Department of Socio-Medical Sciences, Boston University School of Medicine. He received his J.D. from Boston University School of Law in 1973. Among his professional activities, Prof. Glantz is a consultant to the Boston University Center for Health Planning and to the National Center for Health Services Research and is the Associate Editor of *Medicolegal News*. His publications include *Informed Consent to Human Experimentation*, a forthcoming book on *The Rights of Health Care Providers*, and "Decisions Not to Treat: The *Saikewicz* Case and Its Aftermath."

ROBERT J. LEVINE is Professor of Medicine and Lecturer in Pharmacology, Yale University School of Medicine. He received his M.D. from the George Washington University School of Medicine in 1958. Among his diverse professional activities, Dr. Levine is Editor of *IRB: A Review of Human Subjects Research* and a member of the Board of Directors of Medicine In the Public Interest, Inc. He chaired the Department of Medicine's Committee on Policy for Do Not Resuscitate Decisions at Yale–New Haven Hospital and served on the Department of Pediatrics' Committee on Guidelines for Deciding Care of Critically Ill or Dying Patients. Dr. Levine's many publications include a series of papers for the National Commission for the Protection of Human Subjects, which he served as a special consultant from 1974–1978.

PAUL J. LIACOS, Associate Justice of the Massachusetts Supreme Judicial Court, is also Adjunct Professor of Law at Boston University School of Law. He received an LL.B. from Boston University School of Law in 1952 and an LL.M. from Harvard Law School in 1953. Justice Liacos is the author of numerous articles in legal journals and the *Handbook of Massachusetts Evidence*. In November 1977, he delivered the Supreme Judicial Court's opinion in *Superintendent of Belchertown State School* v. *Saikewicz*.

BRUCE L. MILLER is Associate Professor of Philosophy in the Department of Philosophy at Michigan State University, specializing in the philosophy of medicine and law. He received his Ph.D. in Philosophy from Case Western Reserve University in 1970. Prof. Miller's publications include "Open Texture and Judicial Decisions," "Integrating Ethics into the Medical Curriculum," and a report for The Council for Philosophical Studies on Professional

Responsibility in the Law. As a member of the Michigan House of Representatives' Task Force on Death and Dying, he participated in the drafting of that state's Medical Treatment Decision Act.

CATHERINE P. MURPHY is Assistant Professor at the School of Nursing, Boston University; she teaches classes on ethical issues in nursing and is project director of a Department of Health, Education, and Welfare Advanced Training Grant for the preparation of clinical specialists in medical-surgical nursing. She received her M.S. in nursing from Hunter College in 1968 and her Ed.D. from Teachers College, Columbia University, in 1976. Among her professional activities, Prof. Murphy is a member of the Advisory Committee for the Boston University Program in Medicine and Philosophy and of the Massachusetts State Nurses' Association Committee on Ethical Practice. Her publications include "The Moral Situation in Nursing" and a forthcoming volume, *Moral Problems in the Nurse-Patient Relationship.*

MARIANNE PROUT is Head of the Oncology Section at Boston City Hospital and is Assistant Professor in the Departments of Medicine and Socio-Medical Sciences at Boston University School of Medicine. She received her M.D. from Cornell University Medical College in 1971. In addition to publications in the oncology literature, Dr. Prout has developed teaching materials on the dying patient for the Socio-Medical Sciences course at Boston University School of Medicine and has inaugurated both home care and hospice programs for terminally ill cancer patients in inner-city Boston.

JOHN A. ROBERTSON is Associate Professor at the University of Wisconsin Law School and in the Program in Medical Ethics at the University of Wisconsin Medical School. After majoring in philosophy at Dartmouth College, he received his J.D. from Harvard Law School in 1968. Among his professional activities, Prof. Robertson served as a consultant to the National Commission for the Protection of Human Subjects from 1975–1978 and is on the editorial board of *IRB: A Review of Human Subjects Research.* His numerous publications include "Involuntary Euthanasia of Defective Newborns: A Legal Analysis," "Legal Issues in Non-Treatment of Defective Newborns," and *The Rights of the Critically Ill.*

BENSON B. ROE is Professor of Surgery and Co-Chief of Cardiothoracic Surgery at the School of Medicine, University of California, San Francisco. He received his M.D. from Harvard Medical School in 1943. Among his many professional activities, Dr. Roe is a member of the Ethics Committee of the University of California Medical Center, Vice-Chairman of the American Board of Thoracic Surgeons, and a member of the Cardiovascular Committee of the American College of Surgeons. He has written over 100 scientific and clinical articles, including many textbook chapters.

RUSSELL J. ROWELL was President of the Massachusetts Medical Society in 1978–1979 and is currently in private practice in Beverly, Massachusetts, where he is on the staff of Beverly Hospital and President of Beverly Anaesthesia Associates, Inc. He received his M.D. from Tufts University Medical School in 1946. Among his many professional activities, Dr. Rowell serves on the Board of Directors of the New England Academy of Medicine and the Bay State Health Care Foundation, is an executive of the Bay State Professional Standards Review Organization, and is Chairman of the Massachusetts Medical Society's Committee on Legislation.

JUDITH P. SWAZEY is Executive Director of Medicine In the Public Interest, Inc., and Adjunct Professor of Socio-Medical Sciences at Boston University School of Medicine. She received her Ph.D. in the History of Science from Harvard University in 1966. Among her professional activities, Prof. Swazey is a member of the National Academy of Sciences' Institute of Medicine, a fellow of the Institute of Society, Ethics and the Life Sciences, and a consultant to the Office of Technology Assessment, U.S. Congress. Her publications include *Human Aspects of Biomedical Innovation, The Courage to Fail: A Social View of Organ Transplants and Dialysis,* "To Treat or Not to Treat: The Search for Principled Decisions," and "Decisions Not to Treat: The *Saikewicz* Case and Its Aftermath."

I. DAVID TODRES is Director of the Pediatric Intensive Care Unit, Massachusetts General Hospital, a member of the hospital's Critical Care Committee, and Assistant Professor of Anesthesia (Pediatrics) at Harvard Medical School. He received his M.B., Ch.B., from the University of Cape Town, South Africa, in 1958. In 1975, Dr. Todres was the recipient of a National Endowment for the Humanities

Fellowship in Medical Ethics. His publications include "Pediatrics' Attitudes Affecting Decision-Making in Defective Newborns" and a forthcoming textbook, *Intensive Care of the Critically Ill Newborn and Child.*

Introduction

Judith P. Swazey, Ph.D.

> The medicalization of society has brought the epoch of natural death to an end. Western man has lost the right to preside at his act of dying. Health, or the autonomous power to cope, has been expropriated down to the last breath.
>
> Ivan Illich, *Medical Nemesis*

> A dying man needs to die, as a sleeping man needs to sleep, and there comes a time when it is wrong as well as useless to resist. . . . That time has not yet come for me. But it will. It will come for all of us.
>
> Stewart Alsop, *Stay of Execution*

Although death is an inevitable part of nature's life cycle, human beings through the ages have been absorbed with pondering the nature of their mortality. Today, particularly in American society, there is an increasing concern, not with the fact of death, but with the manner of dying. As I write, for example, a quick glance at some of the titles on my bookshelf suggests the flood of "death and dying" literature—popular, sociological, medical-legal, ethical, and religious—that has poured forth in recent years: the *Concern for Dying* newsletter, sections on dying and death in various books on bioethics, and books, to name a few, such as *Euthanasia; Freedom to Die; The Dilemmas of Euthanasia; The Nurse as Caregiver to the Terminal Patient and His Family; Death, Dying, and the Biological Revolution; The Dying Patient; Awareness of Dying; Time for Dying;* and *On Death and Dying.* To works such as these, and others too numerous to mention, we can add as evidence of society's mounting interest in and concern with dying the production of plays, movies, and television shows about the dying patient; a profusion of academic courses on death and dying; training programs for health professionals; and the emergence of careers in "thanatology."[1]

There is no single, simple explanation for this outpouring, which seems to reflect a widespread view of dying as a process fraught with dilemmas for dying individuals, their families and caregivers, and society at large. If there was an event that touched off the past decade's mounting attention to the dying patient, it was the publication in 1969 of Dr. Elisabeth Kübler-Ross's now classic book, *On Death and Dying.* In retrospect, Dr. Kübler-Ross's book was both a causative agent, playing a major role in lifting the public and medical-professional taboo that had shrouded open discussion of dying and death for many decades in America, and a sign of the times, indicating that the dying process presented problems that needed to be acknowledged and addressed visibly.

To enumerate some of these problems briefly, we can begin with sheer numbers. There are some 2 million deaths annually in the United States, and an estimated 1 million persons, at any given time, live with the diagnosis of a terminal illness. These millions as well as the millions who are closely associated with them compose a large "constituency" concerned with the nature of dying in our society. Beyond numbers, advances in medical science and technology have brought about new patterns of morbidity and mortality. Most Americans now die a "slow death," at a later age, from chronic diseases. Over 60 percent of deaths in a given year now occur among persons 65 or older, and there is an increasing time span, an average of 30 months, between a terminal diagnosis and death. Another aspect of the contemporary pattern of dying and death is its location. Most persons today die in a hospital, with over 80 days of hospital care in the year preceding their deaths.

The hospital setting makes dying an increasingly costly process, framing economic, social, and ethical issues about how we ought to allocate health care resources for the terminally ill. In addition, as has been well documented, the nature of the modern hospital as a social system, quite apart from economic factors, all too often makes the time of dying lonely and dehumanized. It is a period of personal and interpersonal stress not only for the dying patient but for family and medical professionals as well.

Another aspect of the modern face of dying, and one most salient to the conference proceedings, is medicine's growing technological capability to sustain life, or depending on one's perspective, to prolong dying. As seen most dramatically in the armamentaria of newborn and adult intensive care units, the occurrence of death can be averted, sometimes indefinitely, by devices and procedures capable of maintaining vital functions.

These technologies have forced us to confront complex and controversial questions about the manner of dying and the event of death: questions about the sanctity of life and the quality of life; about the medical and nonmedical considerations that should enter into decisions on whether or how to treat various types of critical or terminal illnesses and those afflicted with them; about who ought to make such decisions; and about how they ought to be made. Although these questions are given urgency and immediacy by the technology of medicine, they transcend medicine, involving secular and religious values and laws. And the more we ponder them, the more they seem to be true dilemmas, for which no completely or universally satisfactory answers can be found.

As the foregoing suggests, the conference title was chosen deliberately, reflecting our recognition that the issues with which we would be dealing may never be fully resolved, and certainly not in a two-day forum. Our intent, rather, was to bring together a multidisciplinary faculty and participatory audience to explore intensively and attempt to clarify the substantive and procedural dilemmas associated with the care of dying patients. That the conference was held in Boston, as Dr. Farnsworth noted in his preface, was not an accident of time and geography, for the confusion and controversy in Massachusetts that followed in the wake of the *Saikewicz* decision was a major impetus for convoking Dilemmas of Dying.

We were privileged to have the Hon. Paul J. Liacos, author of the *Saikewicz* decision, deliver the keynote address. In his address, speaking publicly about the case for the first time, Justice Liacos reviews the background and content of the decision, discusses misunderstandings and controversies that have ensued since it was handed down in November 1977, and assesses the role of law in the value conflicts surrounding nontreatment decisions.

His address frames the range of medical, legal, social, economic, and ethical issues with which the conference faculty and audience grappled for two days in talks, faculty and audience interchanges, and workshops. Following the conference program, these proceedings are divided into three parts. With some overlap because of their interconnectedness, Parts I and II examine substantive issues in nontreatment decisions, and Part III deals with procedural issues. The chapters in these three parts tend to be informal, because the faculty members were asked to talk to the audience and to each other, rather than, as at most conferences, to read papers. After the presentations at each session, the faculty and audience engaged in often vigorous discussion periods, which are included in these proceedings as edited transcripts.

On a rainy Friday night, half the 200 participants returned for evening workshops—testimony both to their endurance and to their interest in the conference agenda. These workshops, which were not taped for the conference proceedings, dealt with issuing and implementing do not resuscitate orders, nontreatment decisions for critically ill newborns and adults, and judicial and legislative roles in nontreatment decisions. The workshops, their leaders and participants felt, provided a useful small-group format for sharing problems and concerns and for discussing, sometimes heatedly, the differing personal and professional perspectives of the health professionals, lawyers, legislators, judges, and philosophers who were present.

Following Justice Liacos's keynote address, Part I examines nontreatment decisions involving competent adult patients. Chapter 1, by Dr. Robert J. Levine, deals with a recurrently difficult and controversial nontreatment decision: the issuance of do not resuscitate orders. Dr. Levine's talk reviews the approach to deciding on and implementing a do not resuscitate order developed by a Yale–New Haven Hospital policy committee that he chaired. In its report, presented in its entirety in this volume, the policy committee looks at the problems that beset do not resuscitate decisions, such as poor communications between medical and nursing staff and between staff and patients and families, as well as the frequent failure of physicians to think through carefully the objectives of treatment for a given patient. The committee then proposes an authorization scheme, now adopted as official policy by the hospital's medical department, that addresses the medical-technical and the value components of a do not resuscitate decision and offers both substantive and procedural guidelines for making and implementing such decisions.

Oncology is an area of medicine in which the nature of the disease and the state of the art frequently call for decisions by patients and their caregivers about whether to continue active therapeutic intervention. Discussing the measures that she and her staff employ in working out with patients and their families a decision to stop treatment, Dr. Marianne Prout explains in chapter 2 that her major objectives in such decision making are to ascertain the patient's desires and priorities; prevent conflict situations among the staff, patient, and family; and avoid a "Chinese fire-drill syndrome" of all-out medical efforts during the terminal events of a patient's illness. In the majority of cases, she argues, conflicts can and should be resolved without recourse to the courts.

As both Dr. Levine and Dr. Prout recognize, nurses play a central role in caring for and interacting with critically and terminally ill patients, which often places them in stressful situations concerning nontreatment. Chapter 3, by Prof. Catherine P. Murphy, examines within an ethical framework of obligation the dilemmas faced by nurses in nontreatment decisions and outlines the role that she feels nurses should play. Nurses, she maintains, traditionally have had little or no role in making patient care decisions and therefore have the dual problem of implementing nontreatment decisions and facing their ethical and other consequences without having had any voice in the decision itself.

The role and rights of competent patients in nontreatment decisions comprise an area of unsettled, often sharply divergent opinions in medicine, ethics, and the law. In reviewing the law's position on this question, Prof. Leonard H. Glantz finds that the U.S. Supreme Court's 1973 decision in *Roe* v. *Wade* marks a conceptual boundary, the point at which consent and privacy rulings began to advance the proposition that a competent adult does have the right to refuse treatment. No court has said that such refusal is an absolute right, however, and in chapter 4, Prof. Glantz analyzes a series of decisions that set forth possible legal limits to the competent person's right to refuse treatment.

In the discussion following these chapters, the faculty and participants further explore many of the intricate problems surrounding nontreatment decisions for competent adults. Among the topics raised are the legal status of living wills and the legal determination of "competence," a condition that, in clinical settings, often is ambiguous. A converse to the legal and ethical enunciation of the competent patient's right to refuse treatment is the question of how medical staff and families ought to deal with patients who do not want to be informed about or involved in their treatment. Do we want to make patients responsible for making treatment or nontreatment decisions, whether they want to or not? Other questions concern how, legally and in the daily reality of the hospital setting, conflicts are resolved between the wishes of competent dying patients and their families, as well as conflicts among the medical staff. How, legally and morally, can physicians and nurses best handle the conflicts that can arise between what they feel to be their professional responsibilities and the decision-making rights of their patients? As is made clear in the discussion, chapter 5 in this volume, the range of nontreatment decisions that medical professionals and patients face is vast, only hinted at by the extreme cases such as do not resuscitate orders or stopping a respirator. Far more often, medicine involves less dramatic and less publicly visible scenarios, such as decisions about treating an arrhythmia or starting an intravenous line, which are equally demanding of informed thought about the rights and responsibilities of patients and those caring for them.

Arguments about rights and responsibilities in nontreatment decisions grow even more complex as they turn to those who, medically or legally, cannot speak for themselves—incompetent adults and minors. When "voiceless" patients cannot be informed about their prognosis and treatment options and cannot convey their values and wishes, on what bases do we decide whether or how to treat them? And, an inseparable question, who ought to decide? Nowhere are these dilemmas more poignant than in the newborn intensive care unit. In chapter 6, the first selection in part II, Dr. I. David Todres, who directs such a unit, explores the problems of uncertainty surrounding some of the medical criteria employed in making treatment or nontreatment decisions for critically ill newborns. In assessing conditions such as spina bifida, Dr. Todres continues, decisions about whether or how to intervene therapeutically revolve around a concern about the future quality — mental and physical — of the newborn's life. He also points out that quality of life is not a scientifically definable matter, but rather a value judgment that is relative to the person making the judgment.

Granting, as most would, that value-laden judgments about the quality of life are central to treatment or nontreatment decisions, who ought to make such decision for the incompetent patient, and on what kinds of value bases? The answer to the first question, Dr. Benson B. Roe states forcefully in chapter 7, is the physician. Physicians, he argues, have neglected their responsibility for managing human life in jeopardy. It is the physician's duty to determine how patients wish to live, not a buck to be passed to the family or a committee. As part of this duty, Dr. Roe believes, physicians must temper their "crusade to slay the dragon of death" with the realization that humans are not immortal and that resources are limited. The concept of selective treatment or triage, he explains, worked well in wartime, and its principles should be incorporated into civilian medicine.

Judgments about who decides and by what criteria, Prof. Judith P. Swazey suggests, are inextricably linked, and the responses will be shaped by whichever question is addressed first. In chapter 8, she reviews the types of usually ill-defined criteria about the quality of life or value of life that have been used, or advocated, to make nontreatment decisions for incompetent patients in relation to the question of whose best interests such decisions ought to serve. A number of the points raised by Prof. Swazey are also addressed by Prof. John A. Robertson in his examination of the court's role in nontreatment decisions. As illustrated by the *Quinlan, Saikewicz,* and *Dinnerstein* cases, in chapter 9 he analyzes the basic distinction that must be made between substantive and procedural criteria. While the courts seem to be focusing on patient-oriented substantive criteria, Prof.

Robertson finds significant problems in the ways the courts have been applying these criteria.

The discussion session on rights and responsibilities in decision making for incompetent patients underscores the tensions between those who favor such decisions being made by physicians and families and those who feel that, because they are primarily nonmedical value and social policy decisions, they should be made by courts or legislative bodies. The physicians participating in this discussion, chapter 10 in this volume, are themselves ambivalent about these complex questions. On the one hand, for example, several physicians emphasize why a situational decision for each case should be made and stress what they see as the dangers of falling back on "armchair" rule making by those remote from the reality of clinical settings. On the other hand, the physicians also recognize the role that personal and social values play in such decisions and are concerned about physicians assuming that they are best suited to decipher values and act on behalf of an incompetent patient. The leitmotiv of the discussion, setting the stage for part III, is the need for and ability to develop substantive and procedural guidelines.

Turning, in the final session of the conference (Part III), specifically to decision-making procedures, six faculty members present their often divergent perspectives on what procedures are needed and how they might be implemented. Focusing on do not resuscitate procedures, Dr. Russell J. Rowell in chapter 11 assesses the *Dinnerstein* case and its significance for decision making by physicians in relation to the *Saikewicz* case. Prof. Sally Gadow, in turn, offers a perspective grounded in her joint training in nursing and philosophy, in which she examines and rejects paternalism and consumerism as decision-making models. In chapter 12, she proposes an advocacy model in which health professionals actively assist patients in their own decisions and actions, and she then elaborates five themes for establishing advocacy procedures.

From their perspectives as legal scholars, Profs. Robert A. Burt and George J. Annas discuss, respectively, "Immunizing Physicians by Law" and "Learning to Live with Judges." In chapter 13, Prof. Burt challenges what he sees as the desire of physicians to gain complete legal immunity for their actions, holding that they, like patients, must learn to live with uncertainty. He also criticizes decision making by the courts, characterizing it as a highly stylized mode of deliberation often overlooking the human and technological reality of the case being judged and therefore resulting in an irresponsible decision. In chapter 14, meanwhile, Prof. Annas likens the reactions of physicians following the *Saikewicz* decision to the five stages of reactions to dying enunciated by Kübler-Ross; physicians are now in the depression stage. Prof. Annas then presents what he calls a schematic for making nontreatment decisions at different times for competent and incompetent patients, employing medical, legal, and personal criteria.

The final two papers, by Prof. Bruce L. Miller and Sen. Louis P. Bertonazzi, examine legislative roles in establishing procedures for nontreatment decisions. Speaking as a "theorist" rather than as a "strategist," in chapter 15 Prof. Miller reviews the history and content of Michigan's Medical Treatment Decision Act, which he helped draft. Based on the right of competent patients to refuse treatment, the Michigan legislation sets forth provisions for a patient-appointed agent who has the authority to exercise treatment decisions for the patient if the patient becomes incompetent. Sen. Bertonazzi, in contrast, offers a lesson in the reality of legislative politics. In chapter 16, he traces the reasons why, despite mounting concern for some type of living will or right to die legislation, not much has happened or can be expected to happen in the Massachusetts legislature.

Additional concerns and perspectives develop as faculty and participants join in a roundtable discussion of procedural issues and options, which is presented as chapter 17 in this volume. In opening the discussion, Mr. Neil L. Chayet advances a specific procedural proposal, noting that after *Saikewicz*, at least in Massachusetts, "We can't go home again" to traditional modes of private decision making. What Mr. Chayet proposes, and would like to see tested, is the use of a patient representative or surrogate, employed by a hospital, who would have legal or legislative authority to assist competent patients and act on behalf of incompetent patients in treatment or nontreatment decisions.

Following Mr. Chayet's presentation, much of the discussion and debate revolves around questions and suggestions as to why decision making is moving into a legal matrix and, to those who view such a locus as inappropriate, "how we get out of this legal pickle." Themes in this discussion include the merits (or demerits) of legal and legislative procedures and the degree to which courts should be concerned with laying down broad substantive rules for others to follow or with applying rules in individual cases. Although opinions are divided, often sharply, as to who ought to exercise decision-making powers for incompetent patients, there is a common striving to define how the interests of the individual incompetent patient can best be determined and protected.

As the foregoing overview of the conference proceedings implies, the individually written chapters as well as the discussions set forth a wide range of complex, interconnected issues about nontreatment decisions involving both competent and incompetent patients. The substantive and procedural dilemmas faced by all parties engaged in these awesome decisons are numerous, and those attending the conference came away with few definitive answers to their many questions. But the conference did, its organizers believe, succeed in its primary goal: to elucidate more clearly the medical, moral, and legal dilemmas of nontreatment decisions and to expose them to concerned and reasoned inquiry. Most of those who have been involved with nontreatment decisions, I think, would share Dr. Raymond Duff's belief about the "defective" newborn: "the bungling of biology and the limits of power to control it suggest that what is needed is the courage to fail, and that acceptable means should be founded to fail justly and gracefully."[2] How to determine and exercise an "acceptable means" is increasingly a matter of high public concern; and the more such decision making comes out of the closet, the more evident are the substantive and procedural issues that await clarification and resolution.

NOTES

1.   The discussion of the past decade's attention to the dying patient draws extensively on a May 1978 lecture by Dr. Norman A. Scotch in the Boston University School of Medicine's Socio-Medical Sciences course.

2.   R. Duff. A physician's role in decision-making process. In *Decision-making and the defective newborn,* ed. C. A. Swinyard. Springfield, Ill.: Charles C Thomas, 1978, p. 217.

Keynote Address:
The *Saikewicz* Decision*

Hon. Paul J. Liacos

Let me thank you at the outset of this address for the invitation to join with you in exploring the difficult problems that are to be examined over these next two days. I commend the organizers and the various sponsoring organizations for their contribution to the public interest in putting forth a program of this kind. It appears that representatives of both the legal and the medical professions, as well as persons in charge of our great hospitals in this Common-wealth, are joined together in an effort to come to grips with one of the major problems of our day, as reflected in the title of this program: Dilemmas of Dying.

I would think, if I may suggest, respectfully, that the title might well have been Dilemmas of Living, because the problems with which you will all be concerned deal with the decisions that each of us and the patients involved must make in light of new and rapid developments in the field of medical science and medical technology.

---

*The statements contained in this address do not necessarily represent the views of any of the members of the Massachusetts Supreme Judicial Court or express the views of the Massachusetts Supreme Judicial Court.

I confess to feeling a little bit like Daniel, who was cast into the den of the lions, except that I have some doubt whether, like him, I shall survive before this morning is over. Nevertheless, as the person chosen to give the keynote address, I believe it is not my responsibility to discuss the details of the problems with which you will be wrestling in the next two days nor even to try to outline the case law on the subject; I am sure that those particular aspects of your concern will be well handled in the hours to come. Rather, I view my responsibility here in a somewhat different light, namely, to try to present a few key thoughts about which I hope your discussions will revolve. It is my hope also that as a result of this address and this program, all of us from the disciplines of law and medicine and those of us who are in the courts will come to some greater understanding of our respective responsibilities.

Basically, there are three thoughts that I would have you dwell on in connection with your discussions. The first one is that as a result of the *Saikewicz* opinion, a good deal of controversy has taken place. That, I believe, is healthy. What I do not think is necessarily healthy is the fact that a good deal of misinformation has occurred as well, caused both by those not trained in the law and by those who ostensibly claim some degree of medical-legal expertise in the field. It is my hope that this conference will help clarify matters in your mind. The second thought I will seek to address is that one of the fundamental aspects of the *Saikewicz* opinion has been largely overlooked. That is the fact that the interest of the state, sometimes defined under the concept of the so-called *parens patriae* power, has been redefined, so as to recognize the rights of individuals to control their own fates to a much larger extent. Those rights have been guaranteed by *Saikewicz*, not only to the competent, but to incompetent individuals as well. My third thought is perhaps the most controversial one. Through *Saikewicz*, the courts have reasserted, as has been traditionally the case through all areas of social, ethical, and legal significance, their traditional role of safeguarding individual rights by seeing to it that decisions of such great import are made in a principled and public fashion.

Before I discuss each of these areas, let me sketch out the facts of the *Saikewicz* case. The probate court was faced with the problem of a 67-year-old man, a ward of the state, suffering from an acute leukemia; he was profoundly mentally retarded and therefore unable to give informed consent to medical treatment. A guardian ad litem, appointed by the probate court, reported that the illness was incurable, that the only possible treatment was chemotherapy, that such treatment would cause adverse side effects and discomfort and would be incomprehensible to the patient, and that the treatment was not in the patient's best interest. His attending physicians also recommended against chemotherapy. The probate judge subsequently entered an order withholding medical treatment, which the Supreme Judicial Court affirmed.

You may recall that the case commenced when the superintendent of a state institution sought appointment as a temporary and permanent guardian so that chemotherapy could be administered to Mr. Saikewicz. When the state initiated this action, it did so under its so-called *parens patriae* duty to protect an incompetent individual's right to have life-prolonging medical treatment. This remained the position of the Commonwealth throughout the litigation, as represented by the attorney general in his official capacity, acting pursuant to his statutory duty.

One of the less known aspects of the case is that the attorney general was equally active in presenting just the opposite viewpoint. The Civil Rights Division of the Attorney General's Office represented, in part, the interests of Mr. Saikewicz and argued that the chemotherapy treatment should not be administered. Both sides of the state proceeded from different theories. The attorney general stated explicitly, in his brief, that it was the responsibility of the state under its *parens patriae* power to exert every effort to preserve the life of an incompetent individual. The Civil Rights Division, on the other hand, argued that the state's *parens patriae* interest in preserving the life of the incompetent was not sufficient to override or negate the possible exercise of free choice to refuse life-prolonging treatment where appropriate. By its very presence and assertion of that view, the Civil Rights Division recognized the duty of the state to ensure the unfettered exercise of such choice, even in the face of asserted, but ultimately less substantial, state interests. The Civil Rights Division prevailed not only in result, but also in reasoning.

Let me turn now to the first of my thoughts, and that is the unfortunate amount of misinterpretation and misinformation that has arisen from both medical and legal professionals in the field. I need not recount the various articles that have been written as part of the ongoing debate as to the meaning of the *Saikewicz* opinion. Some authors have said that it cast a pall over the medical profession, and indeed one said that it was, in effect, a resounding vote of "no confidence in the medical profession."

I would say that anyone who reads the *Saikewicz* case in that light has entirely misconstrued what was involved factually in the case and has also misconstrued not only the intent but also the language of the opinion. I think that it is true beyond dispute that the factual pattern on which this case was based is one in which the medical professionals involved were entirely in accord that, in the particular circumstances, the treatment commonly called chemotherapy should be withheld, and the court at both the trial and the appellate levels gave every recognition to the value and helpfulness of that medical judgment. Also, the *Saikewicz* opinion emphasized that one of the great interests of the state is the interest of preserving the integrity of the medical profession. How such an opinion could be viewed as a slap at the medical profession is beyond my comprehension. I would suggest that perhaps it reflects more on those who feel criticized than it does on those who allegedly did the criticizing.

As I said, I do not intend to get into an analysis of the various cases. You are all aware of some horrible anecdotes and horrible situations that have been attributed to the *Saikewicz* opinion. I will speak only of one of them, and that is the so-called *Dinnerstein* case, decided by the appeals court. I need not go into a debate about whether *Dinnerstein* is technically in accord with *Saikewicz* or not; that is not my point in raising this issue at this time. What I will simply say is that *Dinnerstein* strikes me as a case that need never have been litigated, because it was clearly not within the scope of *Saikewicz*. For hospitals to be advised that a do not resuscitate order could not be instituted and that a person who was terminally ill had to be resuscitated time and time again in the absence of legal and judicial determination is an entirely misleading interpretation of the *Saikewicz* opinion. The *Saikewicz* case, after all, upheld the witholding of chemotherapy, treatment that might very well have prolonged the life of Joseph Saikewicz for a number of months. Thus, I can only say, without necessarily accepting the reasoning of the appeals court in this matter, that the result there in my view was wholly consistent with what was stated in the *Saikewicz* case. I speak, of course, for myself and not for my colleagues, but I cannot help but repeat that *Dinnerstein* seems to me to have been an example not only of an abundance of caution but of hysteria on the part of legal counsel who advised the hospital to take such extreme measures in order to protect the hospital and the medical staff.

This leads me to another thought, and I am not alone in expressing it. If the medical profession seeks to be immunized with certainty from each and every possible claim, civil or ciminal, then that is one thing, but let us not confuse that desire as being a motive involving the best interest of the patient. While such immunity strikes me as a legitimate concern, it serves to protect the hospital and the medical staff rather than the interest of the patient. If that is what the medical profession feels it must have, then I would suggest that perhaps *Saikewicz* is a boon because, if you want to interpret it that way, you can get a predetermination of your rights rather than suffer the risk of having a hindsight determination in which you might be held to have acted improperly. I raise this thought merely to point out that there is a difference between acting to preserve the interest of the patient and acting to preserve the interest of the profession. I am sorry to say that, to me, the lawyers in the *Dinnerstein* case seemed to be acting on the latter rather than on the former.

In short, the court has recognized and has every confidence in the integrity and competence of the medical profession. To say that the court has a role to play in certain of these areas is not a slap at the medical profession; it is an indication of willingness to work cooperatively with the medical profession in an effort to help resolve some of the most difficult problems of our day.

Let me next turn to the concept of state power that is involved in *Saikewicz*. A clear reading of this opinion, it seems to me, is that for the first time the court in this Commonwealth recognized the right of persons to act reasonably and rationally in regard to whether or not they wished to undertake a course of medical treatment. In so doing, the court rejected, in effect, the traditional *parens patriae* approach that the interest of the state, particularly its interest in the preservation of life, will always and without qualification prevail against the interest of individuals to make their own choices as to what they want done with their bodies and their fates.

The state traditionally has claimed four interests: (1) the preservation of life, (2) the protection of interests of third parties, (3) the prevention of suicide, and (4) the maintenance of the ethical integrity of the medical profession. Under existing legal doctrines before *Saikewicz*, these four interests have been arrayed against an individual's informed decision to decline medical treatment. Before *Saikewicz*, the state, through its public officers, was committed to an affirmance of abstract and attenuated state interest in life against the concrete particulars of an individual's decision, actual or imputed, to accept or decline medical treatment.

In recognizing the force of the individual's rights against the state interests asserted, and in imposing on the state the duty to protect the exercise and existence of the individual's rights, *Saikewicz* fundamentally redefined the relationship of state and individual. If, before *Saikewicz*, the state interest in preserving life was always deemed to override the individual's actual or imputed decision, that is no longer true. Rather, now the individual's desires may be of equal or greater magnitude. The protection of the individual's right to accept or reject life-prolonging treatment is now a separate and independent state interest, to be added to those traditionally used to circumscribe the individual's freedom of choice.

The question then arises as to what this philosophical change means in practical terms. If freedom of choice is now a state interest to be protected, the state has as much obligation to enforce the individual's right to have that freedom of choice as it has, in the view of the attorney general, to enforce its interests in preserving life. If efforts are being made to infringe the rights of an incompetent individual in its custody to refuse medical treatment, it is the obligation of the state to protect that individual's freedom of choice from such interference. Correlatively, the state is obligated to provide life-prolonging treatment where the individual choice is consistent with such a position. The state must vigorously protect not only the right to decline but also the right to accept medical treatment. The individual's freedom to decide the fundamental questions involving privacy and bodily integrity must be protected.

That is one reason why the fact that the judiciary now may

be involved in these decisions is not only appropriate but indeed necessary. It is traditionally the function of the judiciary to protect individuals against unwarranted exercises of state power. The judiciary must ensure that the state's actions involving individuals are consistent with the limitations on its power as well as with a respect for the integrity of individual rights. If, as I suggest we should, we view *Saikewicz* as redefining the relationship between individual and state, then the only forum that has the competence, stature, and authority to protect individual rights from state infringement is the judiciary. The judiciary is the only institution sufficiently disinterested to permit a neutral yet binding resolution to such controversies. Of course, not every medical decision requires a lawsuit. However, some life-and-death decisions are so fraught with difficulties that the due process and procedural safeguards of the judicial system are necessary to protect the rights of patients, relatives, physicians, and state officers.

Last, let me suggest an alternative justification for what some have viewed as the intrusion of the courts into this area, and this is the fact that many of the questions that physicians face on the front lines every day can no longer be viewed solely as medical questions. At the outset, I suggested that perhaps this conference should have been called Dilemmas of Living. You are all aware, even more than I, of the fantastic range of new knowledge and technology in the area of medical science. Our society today, and for some recent years, has been struggling to redefine its views on the meaning of life and death, on when life starts and when it ends, on what can be done by the use of implanted organs or transplanted organs, on problems of abortion, on problems of genetic engineering, and on the use of new technologies now available to maintain and perhaps, in the not-too-distant future, even create life.

To suggest that these questions are wholly medical questions is to overlook the concerns not only of the judiciary and of the legal profession, but of the public as well. Indeed, within the medical profession, the recent proliferation of persons specializing in these issues—not just from the point of view of medicine, but also from the point of view of ethics, philosophy, morality, and law—reflects the recognition that many of these questions, albeit not all, have the deepest implications for the well-being of our society. To say that the courts have no role in this area is not only to rebuff what might be viewed by some as a chauvinistic attempt by the judiciary to insert itself into an area into which it has never ventured before. Such a view challenges not the courts, but the very nature of our society. Questions of life and death, of morality and ethics, and of individual rights have been traditional concerns of the courts in a wide variety of human endeavors. To say that the medical profession stands alone, apart from the scientists, the nuclear engineers, and the technicians and experts in every other field, and that it must be unsupervised and unfettered in its activities, is to deny, I think, the very principles on which our society has been founded.

What the court is saying in *Saikewicz* is that questions of life and death are not purely medical questions and not purely questions of science and technology; rather, they are questions involving ethical, social, and moral considerations, as well as medical and legal considerations. This traditionally has been the place where the courts most meaningfully have had a role in regulating the development of our society in our democracy.

I would suggest also that the *Saikewicz* decision, in causing the controversy it has, should be viewed as a healthy beginning, not as an end and not as the be-all and end-all to this question. The fact that we are here today in mutual discussion, seeking to join together to understand the problems that face us, is indeed a most healthy sign. The courts can bring to this area most of the characteristics of the rule of law that I think all might agree have been some of the proudest characteristics of our society. We need the help of the medical profession. We are willing and anxious to work with that profession, but what needs to be done is to have principled decision making open to public scrutiny by persons impartial to the process of decision making and in a forum in which all points of view and all facts can be developed. In saying this, I recognize the limitations of the judicial system and its processes. But I would add that unless we are all willing to have these life-and-death decisions made in such a forum, we would then be faced with the claim that matters of life and death are privately being made without regulation, without oversight of the public interest, and without adequate protection of the interest of the most crucial parties involved, namely, patients and their families. Nor would we be protecting the interests of the state in these very delicate matters.

I am sympathetic, although you may not think so, to the

concerns of physicians. As a judge, I have similar feelings that it would be much nicer to be able to make my decisions without being subjected to the public analysis, criticism, and debate to which this one opinion of mine has been subjected. I live daily under such scrutiny. In human terms, I would prefer not to have this happen. In professional terms, and as a responsible citizen, I welcome it, and I hope that you will join me in welcoming this ongoing debate concerning one of the most significant parts of our social problems. I am mindful in saying this that some of you may not accept it easily. I am also mindful that the courts work on a case-by-case basis, and no one decision can answer all the problems involved, nor even adequately define the parameters of the problem.

Saikewicz, as I have said, is not the end of this problem. It is, I think, a healthy beginning, in that it brought this kind of question out into the open. To the extent that we are talking about not only the rights of the competent, but the rights of the incompetent as well, it is particularly important that our society face up to its responsibilities to people unfortunately afflicted with such problems as was Joseph Saikewicz. Value judgments, yours and mine, are always involved in decision making, whether we think they are or not. The best way to come to grips with problems of this kind is to start on the process and to work together to try to bring about a procedure and a way of decision making that will accommodate all the conflicting interests involved.

Despite what I have indicated as being misinterpretations of *Saikewicz*, I remain hopeful that this process is now well under way, and if *Saikewicz* has caused each and every one of us to discuss openly the major issues of life and death in modern society, then I would rest my case and say that *Saikewicz* has been successful.

THE COMPETENT PATIENT AND RIGHTS TO REFUSE TREATMENT

I

Do Not Resuscitate Decisions and Their Implementation

Robert J. Levine, M.D.

1

At the conference, I presented a paper entitled "The Authorization of Do Not Resuscitate Orders by Patients and Families." Much of the presentation was drawn from a March 1979 report prepared by the Committee on Policy for Do Not Resuscitate Decisions, an ad hoc committee of the Department of Medicine of Yale–New Haven Hospital.[1] Since many participants at the conference expressed interest in this report, it is published here in place of my original presentation. But first, a few introductory remarks.

Perhaps the single most important feature of this report is that it calls on the responsible physician to identify the objectives of management of any patient who either is or appears to be terminally ill. This identification is done according to a management classification scheme, which is given in the third section, "Classification of Approaches to Management of the Terminally Ill." The overall objective may be (1) to produce a cure or remission, (2) to maintain biological function, or (3) to comfort patients as they are dying. In the process of identifying the management objectives for any particular patient, the responsible physician is forced to confront the fact that therapeutic maneuvers designed to advance one of these objectives will often be detrimental to one or both of the other objectives. For example, maneuvers performed to increase the likelihood of cure will commonly produce discomfort, undermine biological function, or both. Formal identification of the overall management objective frequently has heuristic value. It may expose to members of the health care team the fact that some of their activities are incompatible with their objectives. Consequently, they may reconsider and modify either their activities or their objective.

This report makes no provision for the development of committees to review do not resuscitate decisions. We considered and rejected the concept of an "ethics" committee, as mandated in New Jersey by the *Quinlan* decision. Our judgment was that the health care team that is working with a particular patient should be presumed to be the most expert "ad hoc prognosis committee" that could be convened under the circumstances. In the second section, "Communications among Health Care Professionals," the responsible physician is charged to cause this ad hoc committee to take timely and appropriate action; in addition, some rules of procedure are provided.

The fourth section, "Communications with the Patient and Family," presents some of the ways in which patients and their families may express and actuate their choices about management. In general, health professionals are urged to initiate discussion of such choices early in the course of the patient's disease, when the patient is most capable of meaningful participation in such discussion. However, it is acknowledged that in a hospital setting, these discussions often are not initiated until it seems appropriate to discontinue attempts to produce cures or remissions.

In some circumstances, patients or their relatives are asked for authorization of (not informed consent to) a shift in the objectives of management from curing to either maintaining function or maximizing comfort. Requests for authorization are appropriate when the discussion is initiated by the responsible physician because, in the judgment of the health care team, there is no chance of medical reversibility of the basic disease process (these terms are defined in the third section under the heading, "Definitions," on pages 31–34). Therefore, it is not appropriate to ask the patient or the relatives whether they wish to attempt curative therapy. More precisely, they are called on to acknowledge that death is inevitable. Under these conditions, we do not recommend aspiring to a condition that might properly be termed "informed consent." Clear statements of risks, benefits, alternatives, and so on, do not—in these circumstances—foster the patient's autonomy. Rather, such discussions impose on patients and their relatives the burden of having to make decisions that are not truly theirs to make.

At the time of this writing (August 1979), the following report is the official policy of the Department of Medicine at Yale–New Haven Hospital. Its suitability for other departments remains to be determined by the hospital's governing board. This policy is compatible with legal requirements of the state of Connecticut; in other jurisdictions, different procedures may be required by state law.

REPORT OF THE COMMITTEE
ON POLICY FOR
DO NOT RESUSCITATE DECISIONS

The committee concludes that the most important obstacle to the making and implementation of decisions on withholding cardiopulmonary resuscitation is faulty communications. Some of the more important barriers to communication in the current system are discussed next:

1. It is sometimes difficult to identify the responsible physician, the individual who has the responsibility for seeing to it that decisions are made, communicated, and implemented. This is particularly true in the intensive care unit when multiple subspecialists are involved in the management of a patient.

2. Some members of the health care team who have important information that is germane to a decision may not make that information available to the responsible physician because (a) they are unaware that a decision is to be made or (b) some nonphysicians—for example, nurses or social workers—feel that they may be perceived as overstepping their bounds if they initiate discussions of such decisions with physicians.

3. Some physicians believe incorrectly that writing a do not resuscitate order will increase the likelihood of malpractice litigation. In fact, writing such orders in accord with the recommendations of this report will have the opposite effect.

4. Discussions between the responsible physician and the patient are at times initiated much too late. Discussions initiated in the suboptimal conditions of the intensive care unit often could have been anticipated by several months and conducted in a much more satisfactory setting.

5. The authority to accept or refuse resuscitation (or any other therapeutic maneuver) properly resides with the patient or the next of kin. The physician, on the other hand, is most capable of predicting the consequences of any therapeutic intervention. In some cases, there are great differences between what the patient wishes and what the physician judges to be possible; such differences are likely to be associated with unsatisfactory communication.

6. In some cases in which a decision has been made to withhold resuscitation (or any other therapeutic maneuver), not all health professionals who might come into contact with the patient are aware of it. Consequently, such interventions may be performed when they are contrary to the expressed will of

the patient. Parenthetically, this seems to be an uncommon experience at Yale–New Haven Hospital.

This report reflects the committee's attempt to eradicate—or at least to minimize—the six specified barriers to communication; other barriers perceived by the committee are implicit in our recommendations for dealing with them. This report provides no guidelines for determining what medical conditions are to be considered grounds for withholding resuscitation or other life-sustaining therapy. Rather, it identifies the personnel who should be held accountable for ensuring that such decisions are made and the procedures that they should employ to facilitate clear and unambiguous communications relevant to these decisions.

The recommendations are presented in the following order:

   I. Identification of the responsible physician
  II. Communications among health care professionals
 III. Classification of approaches to management of the terminally ill
 IV. Communications with the patient and family
  V. The mechanics of writing do not resuscitate orders and classification notes

I. Identification of the responsible physician

In March 1978, the Medical Board and the Board of Directors of the Yale–New Haven Hospital approved an updated version of the "Policies Governing Responsibility for Care of Patients" in the hospital. These policies specify that all patients admitted to Yale–New Haven Hospital are to be under the care of a member of the hospital staff who is designated as the "responsible physician." The responsible physician has the overall responsibility, both medically and legally, for the patient's care. A detailed account of the duties of the responsible physician can be found in the policy statement.

In the care of patients who are terminally ill, clear identification of the responsible physician is of paramount importance. If at any time the identity of the responsible physician is unclear to any member of the health care team, he or she should ask the house officer to identify the responsible physician. If the house officer is unable to do so, he or she should contact the chief medical resident, who has the obligation to provide a prompt identification of the responsible physician.

The obligations of the responsible physician in the care of terminally ill patients—in addition to those specified in the Yale–New Haven Hospital policies—are as follows:

1. Coordination of communications among various members of the health care team and with various professional consultants.
2. Communication with the patient, the family, or both, with the aim of seeking an agreement to a specific management classification with or without a do not resuscitate order.
3. Writing of the management classification with or without a do not resuscitate order in the chart.
4. In cases of irreconcilable disagreement, activation of the appeals mechanism (cf. Section II).

II. Communications among health care professionals

Although the ultimate responsibility for medical decision making rests with the responsible physician, other members of the health care team often have important information that they might be able to contribute to the decision-making process. In order to ensure access to all relevant information at the time of making decisions about management classifications as well as do not resuscitate orders, the committee makes the following recommendation:

> When it becomes apparent to the responsible physician that a decision must be made about management classification of a terminally ill patient, the physician should signal to all members of the health care team the intention to make such a decision by writing a note to that effect in the patient's chart. Such a note might be worded: "The condition of this patient is deteriorating and it is necessary to formulate plans with regard to future managment. This will be done at (specify a time and place; e.g., tomorrow at work rounds)."

Such a note should alert all parties (e.g., physicians, nurses, social workers, chaplains, and students) that a management classification decision is about to be made. In this way, they are alerted to contribute any information they consider relevant to the decision-making process. They may either speak directly with the responsible physician or the house officer or they might plan to be present at the designated time for making the decision.

In general, health care personnel should refrain from initiating discussions with the patient or the family that seem to reflect a consensus on management classification until such a consensus is reached through appropriate discussions among members of the health care team.

It is a strong conviction of the committee that any member of the health care team who considers that the management classification for a patient is inappropriate (or, in some cases, when there is no management classification, that there should be one) should report this opinion to the responsible physician; any health care professional holding such an opinion should consider it an obligation, not merely a prerogative, to report such an opinion to the responsible physician. Furthermore, it is the obligation of the responsible physician to act upon such communications. The responsible physician has the right and the obligation to make final judgments about the medical reversibility (defined in the next section) of the patient's condition; in the event of irreconcilable disagreements among health care professionals, suitable consultation should be obtained. If the disagreements cannot be resolved with the aid of a consultant, the matter should be referred to the chief of service for arbitration or mediation.

In many instances, the physician having the best relationship with the family or the patient may be a member of the house staff and not the responsible physician. Therefore, discussions with the patient or family that ultimately lead to a change in management classification (with or without a do not resuscitate order) may be conducted by that member of the house staff. However, these discussions should first be approved by the responsible physician; delegation of authority to conduct such discussions must be explicit.

The authority to write a do not resuscitate order may not be delegated; it must be written personally by the responsible physician. However, house officers have the authority to cancel do not resuscitate orders as appropriate. For example, such orders should be canceled at the request of the patient or duly authorized member of the family (cf. Section IV). In addition, an unexpected finding that suggests that the prognosis for medical reversibility has been substantially underestimated should signal the need for cancellation of a do not resuscitate order. In the latter case, the order should be suspended temporarily while the house officer attempts to discuss the unexpected finding with the responsible physician.

In the absence of a house officer, nurses may be called upon by family members to perform cardiopulmonary resuscitation on patients for whom do not resuscitate orders have been written. Under these circumstances, the nurse should contact either the house officer or the responsible physician as soon as possible. In the event the request to disregard a do not resuscitate order is made during cardiopulmonary arrest and no physician is available, the nurse is authorized to proceed with cardiopulmonary resuscitation. However, all professionals should be aware that—at the moment of cardiopulmonary arrest—members of the family who have previously carefully thought through decisions to authorize do not resuscitate orders may respond to the immediate situation by saying, "Do something." Professionals who are experienced at working in intensive care units can ordinarily distinguish this reaction from a determination to reverse a previously well-thought-out decision. Commonly, at such times, the family member is more in need of attention than the patient.

III. Classification of approaches to management of the terminally ill

When patients either are or appear to be terminally ill, some members of the health care team may not have clear understandings of the team's overall management objectives. In some cases, this is because these objectives have not been defined by the responsible physician; the necessary consultations and discussions may not yet have been accomplished.

In other cases, the objectives may be clear to the responsible physician but not clearly articulated to others who should be aware of them. In the absence of clear articulation of overall objectives, there is the ever-present possibility that a health care professional might either initiate or withhold a therapeutic maneuver and, by so doing, undermine the mangement objectives.

In this section, we present a system for classification of overall management objectives. The purpose of this classification system is to provide an easily accessible reference for those health professionals who might be called upon to make judgments about implementing various therapeutic maneuvers when the responsible physician is not available for timely consultation.

Class A: The general presumption in this class is that patients are to receive all curative and functional maintenance therapies* as indicated. The primary goal is to achieve arrest, remission, or cure of the basic disease process. The aims of curative therapy take priority over those of functional maintenance, which, in turn, hold a higher priority than those of comforting therapy.

Class B: The general presumption in this class is that any curative therapy in progress (if any) will be continued until its outcome has been determined and, further, no new curative therapy will be implemented. The goals of functional maintenance therapy take priority over the goals of comforting therapy. The responsible physician should specify limits—if any—to be imposed on functional maintenance therapy (e.g., if sepsis occurs, should it be treated with antibiotics?).

Class B is further subdivided as follows:

B1: In the event of cardiopulmonary arrest, the patient is to be resuscitated.

B2: A do not resuscitate order is written.

Class C: The goals of therapy are to comfort the patient as he or she is dying. A do not resuscitate order is written, and comforting therapy dominates the approach to medical care. The limits of functional maintenance therapy should be specified.

Definitions

Basic disease process: This is the disease process that plays the dominant role in determining whether or not the patient's illness is "medically reversible" (*infra*). In some patients, there may be two (or, rarely, more) basic disease processes.

Medical reversibility: The medical reversibility of a basic disease

---

* Definitions of these classes of therapy are provided subsequently in this section.

process is strictly a technical judgment. In the hospital setting, the personnel who are most qualified to render such a judgment are physicians. Judgments with regard to medical reversibility should include statements both of its probability and of its magnitude. A characteristic technical statement of medical reversibility is as follows—if we implement therapy X, there is about a 10-percent chance of inducing a 50-percent reduction in, for example, the size of the tumor. In order to translate this technical statement into language that is of use to a patient and the patient's family, an elaboration is ordinarily required. For example, if we implement therapy X, there is about a 10-percent chance that it will work. If it does, we might hope to see a substantial return of, e.g., cognitive function.

Curative therapy: These are therapies that are directed at the basic disease process for the purpose of either arresting or reversing its progress, with the aim of inducing a partial or total remission. Implementation of a curative therapy presupposes that a judgment has been made and that the basic disease process is potentially medically reversible.

Functional equilibrium: This term refers to a physiological status of the patient that is compatible with biological survival. In general, a patient is said to be in functional equilibrium if adequate ventilation, nutrition, perfusion of vital organs, excretory function, and so on, are present. Impairments of any of these functions may be caused by a variety of phenomena that may or may not be labeled appropriately as diseases. For example, impairments in respiratory function might be caused by obstruction to the airways either by excessive secretions or by tumors. They may also be caused by pneumonia or by paralysis of respiratory muscles. Actions directed toward removing these detriments to respiratory function are performed in the interests of maintaining functional equilibrium, notwithstanding the status of the detriment as a disease or something else.

Pneumonia, for example, may be viewed as either a basic disease process or as a detriment to functional equilibrium. Its status is determined by virtue of its role in making global determinations of the potential reversibility of the patient's medical illness. Thus, in a patient having a basic disease process—e.g., a metastatic solid tumor—that has rendered him or her totally incapacitated and that—in the considered judgment of the health care team—is nearly devoid of potential for medical reversibility, treatment of pneumonia may be considered functional maintenance therapy. A decision to treat pneumonia in such a patient has much more in common with a decision to use a respirator than it does with a decision to administer so-called curative therapy.

Functional maintenance therapy: These are therapies designed to achieve or maintain functional equilibrium.

Comforting therapy: These are therapies designed to achieve or maintain the patient's comfort.

Determinations of what constitutes functional equilibrium lie almost exclusively in the domain of the physician. By contrast, when the patient is capable of communicating, determinations of what constitutes comfort lie exclusively in his or her domain. Often, therapies designed to be curative or to maintain functional equilibrium (e.g., endotracheal tubes) will produce discomfort. Similarly, therapies designed to produce comfort may induce functional disequilibria (e.g., morphine given for purposes of producing comfort may inhibit respiratory function or induce ileus). Thus, it is necessary to make clear statements as to whether producing comfort takes priority over maintaining functional equilibrium.

Although the patient or the physician may be most competent to make judgments as to what constitutes comfort or functional equilibrium, respectively, such judgments are to be distinguished from decisions to take action. Decisions to take actions (e.g., implementation or withholding of various therapeutic maneuvers) are to be done in accord with agreements reached through appropriate discussions among all concerned parties—health care professionals and patients or their families, or both.

The general presumption is that all patients are in Class A unless otherwise specified. Patients are to be classified according to this system only when there exists some legitimate cause to suspect that a patient should be in either Class B or C. Writing in the chart that a patient is in Class A should be done only to signal the fact that the health care team has—with due deliberation and consultation—rejected classifying the patient as either B or C.

Patients should be classified in Class B only when there is a very low probability of achieving any consequential remission. In general, reasonable curative therapies would have already been tried and have failed or would have been rejected for good cause. For example, the patient may have refused some potentially curative therapies. For some patients in this class, a curative therapy may be in progress but there is little likelihood of success.

Class B is, in general, to be considered a temporary classification. Some of these patients will show surprising responses to curative therapy, in which case they will be transferred to Class A. Most of them, however, will become suitable candidates for Class C.

IV. Communications with the patient and family

When the responsible physician—with due consultation with other health care professionals—has reached a decision with regard to the medical reversibility of a patient's condition, a discussion should be initiated with the patient or the family, or both, with the aim of defining the overall management objectives. The ultimate authority to determine the overall management objectives resides with the patient or the family; this is elaborated subsequently in this section. The discussions should ordinarily be conducted by the responsible physician; however, when appropriate, this responsibility may be delegated to a house officer (cf. Section II).

If the patient is conscious and competent, he or she has the clear right to refuse any treatment (including resuscitation) even if the consequences of such refusal may be death. Thus, if the patient, after discussion of the alternatives, is capable of understanding the situation and wishes not to be resuscitated, the physician is entitled to rely on such a decision; this entitlement obtains even when the decision is opposed by one or more of the patient's relatives. In general, if a competent adult patient refuses any therapy, the therapy may be given only when authorized by a court order. It should be noted, however, that in cases of attempted suicide, it is customary and legal to oppose the expressed wishes of the patient to refuse lifesaving therapy.

If a legally competent patient is steadfast in refusing any type of therapy and if in the judgment of the responsible physician, such refusal seems irrational, the chief of staff or hospital counsel should be consulted. It should be noted that the hospital will almost never initiate incompetency proceedings based solely on the fact that a patient is refusing treatment.

If the patient is comatose or incompetent and a legal guardian (known in Connecticut as the conservator of the person) has been appointed, the conservator of the person has the right to make such decisions. Only a patient who has been so adjudicated by a court is legally incompetent; all other patients are to be considered competent as a matter of law. Ideally, the family should be urged to obtain a court order appointing a conservator prior to the time such decisions are to be made if the patient seems incapable of speaking for himself or herself; however, in many cases, this action is impractical.

Decisions to discontinue lifesaving therapies or to withhold resuscitation must be authorized by the patient or, when appropriate, the guardian. Failure to secure such authorization may impose legal liability on the physician. Consequently, when such decisions are contemplated in the course of management of comatose or incompetent patients, every effort should be made to contact an individual who is entitled to provide such authorization. If such a person cannot be located, the chief of staff and hospital counsel should be notified.

If the patient is comatose or legally incompetent, the following order of decision making should be followed. The spouse, if present and competent, has the clear paramount right over adult children to be appointed conservator of an incompetent patient and, even if not appointed, to make decisions about treatment. If there is no spouse but there are adult offspring, if there is consensus among the siblings, any one sibling may act for all. If there is disagreement, hospital counsel should be called.

When the authority to make a decision resides in a group (e.g., of siblings), it is legally perilous to discontinue therapy while there is conflict among members of the group. At times it may be necessary to resuscitate the patient, perhaps several times, while awaiting consensus to develop.

Some legally incompetent patients may be capable of expressing their wishes about their management. When there are conflicts between the conservator and the patient, no decision to withdraw curative or functional maintenance therapies or to write do not resuscitate orders should be made without authorization from the chief of staff and the hospital counsel.

In any case in which the physician believes there is a reasonable possibility of medical reversibility of the basic disease process and the patient is comatose or incompetent, the physician has the legal authority to treat the patient over the family's objection. One should be aware of the possibility of conflicts of interest between a terminally ill patient and his or her relatives. In the event a family member is adamant in opposing a physician's plans to continue life-sustaining therapy, hospital counsel should be consulted.

In some cases in which the responsible physician and the patient or family, or both, are in irreconcilable conflict about the appropriate course of management, the physician may offer to withdraw. In these circumstances, the responsible physician should also offer assistance in identifying and contacting another physician who will assume the role of responsible physician.

According to Yale–New Haven Hospital policy, therapeutic procedures should be implemented only with the informed consent of the patient. The agreements reached between physicians and patients or their families, or both, that result in management classifications with or without do not resuscitate orders may, at times, be based on discussions that can truly be considered as resulting in a condition known as "informed consent." In general, this term can be properly applied in cases where the discussions are begun several weeks or months before a do not resuscitate order might be implemented. In such cases, the negotiations for informed consent may result in a document known as a "living will." The committee strongly encourages the early initiation of such discussions and the development of living wills. Such documents provide the most clear and unambiguous expressions of the patients' values rendered at times when the patients are relatively rational and autonomous and when there is time for due deliberation; their situations are substantially and relevantly different from what they will be in the intensive care unit.

When discussions are initiated by physicians under circumstances in which it seems appropriate to enter a patient in management Class B or C, it is rarely possible to achieve informed consent. Ordinarily, the physician approaches the patient or family, or both, with a statement that there is no reasonable chance of medical reversibility; accordingly, they are asked to "authorize" a shift in management objectives to Class B or C. The committee recommends that the term "authorization" be used to refer to such agreements. As much time and support should be given as is necessary for the patient or family, or both, to reach a decision and to seek consultation with such advisors as they may choose, medical and otherwise. In these cases, what is sought is the authorization of the patient or the family to a particular plan of management based on the estimation of the health care professionals as to what medicine can and cannot achieve. However, the patient or family, or both, has the legal authority to require that a patient be managed according to Class B1 even when the physican believes that Class C management would be more appropriate; the physician is obliged to proceed according to these wishes.

In the event a patient meets the criteria* for "brain death," the patient may be pronounced dead and then all therapeutic maneuvers may be discontinued, notwithstanding any expressions of wishes to do otherwise.

V. The mechanics of writing do not resuscitate orders and classification notes

Decisions to withhold resuscitation in the event of cardiopulmonary arrest are to be written on the order sheet. They should be spelled out; the abbreviation DNR should not be used. Also not to be used are such euphemisms as "No code" or "In case of CPA, page house officer, stat." Only the responsible physician may write the do not resuscitate order. It is presumed that do not resuscitate orders will be reviewed at least once daily and commonly more frequently. The committee considered and rejected recommending that these orders have automatic expiration periods, for example, 24 hours.

According to Yale–New Haven Hospital policies, all orders are to be written. In emergencies, it is acceptable for physicians to

---

*See: Black, P. M. Brain death. *N. Engl. J. Med.* 299:338–344 and 393–401, 1978.

give oral orders for therapeutic actions other than do not resuscitate orders. Usually, oral orders are appropriate in emergencies when it would be detrimental to the interests of the patient to wait for orders to be written. This justification is never appropriate for do not resuscitate orders; they must always be written.

The committee recommends that the physician write on the order sheet a notification that a management classification note has been written in the progress notes. This note should indicate the date on which it was written and identify the individual who wrote it. Substantive changes in the management classification should also be similarly noted on the order sheet.

In all cases in which a do not resuscitate order is written, a management classification note is mandatory.

In the Kardex, the nurse should note prominently that a do not resuscitate order has been written. In close proximity to this notation, there should be an additional notation of when the most current management classification note was written in the progress notes. When applicable, there should also be a list of limitations of such things as functional maintenance therapies.

Progress notes: Management classification notes should provide a clear account of the rationale for the determination of the objectives of management. There should be an identification of the basic disease process or processes and an estimation of the probability and magnitude of its medical reversibility. There should be a statement as to whether the management objectives are those of Class A, B (1 or 2), or C. Limitations, if any, on functional maintenance therapies (or other therapies) that have been agreed upon with the patient are to be identified. Further, there should be a statement about the extent to which the objectives of comforting take priority over those of functional maintenance.

Finally, there should be a statement as to who authorized this approach to management—either the patient or the appropriate relative(s) or guardian. This statement should include a brief account of the information that was conveyed to the patient or family, or both, that formed the basis of the authorization.

In general, a competent patient should not be asked to document authorization of a do not resuscitate order when it appears that there might soon be a need for its implementation.

Such a request might be considered appropriate following thorough discussions of the matter several weeks or months before it appears that the do not resuscitate order might be implemented. Ordinarily, in the early stages of an inevitably fatal disease, it is preferable to suggest to the patient that he or she might wish to develop a living will; if the patient wishes, a copy of this document may be put in the chart.

Occasionally, it is necessary to ask either the patient or a member of the family to sign an authorization note for a do not resuscitate order. These are situations in which either (1) there is irreconcilable disagreement between the person having the legal authority to make the decision and one or more members of the family or (2) strong disagreements between equally entitled siblings have recently been resolved. In these cases, the member of the family who takes responsibility for authorizing a do not resuscitate order should be asked to sign (or, if preferred, write) an authorization note in the medical record (progress notes). This should be a brief note indicating that the responsible person(s) understands and agrees to the do not resuscitate order. The note should include the fact that the condition of the patient is terminal, that discussions have been held with the family (and, if appropriate, with the patient), and that a decision has been made not to resuscitate that patient in the event that breathing or the heart stops. Although no set form for such a note is suggested by the committee, each note should include a reasonably full statement of the rationale for the decision and a summary of the discussions with the patient or family. Those who prefer not to sign such notes should not be coerced to do so; in such cases, the physician should record the fact that the individual(s) preferred not to sign the note; the reasons for this preference, if known, should also be recorded.

It is of utmost importance that the existence of a do not resuscitate order be communicated effectively to all members of the health care team. It should not be difficult to ensure awareness of such orders on the part of those health care personnel who are assigned to work on various shifts in the patient care unit. Occasionally, patients for whom do not resuscitate orders are written are transported to other parts of the hospital to receive a diagnostic or therapeutic service. Thus, they may come into contact with health professionals who will be unaware of the do not resuscitate order unless appropriate precautions are taken. Therefore, the committee recommends that it be made the obligation of the responsible physician (or the house officer to whom he or she delegates such responsibility) to communicate clearly with the personnel of the department (e.g., the x-ray department) to which the patient is being transported that there is a do not resuscitate order. Ideally, a professional from the patient care unit should accompany the patient to make sure that—among other things—do not resuscitate orders are respected. When this is not feasible, however, the responsible physician—or the physician's delegate—should communicate clearly to a health professional in the department to which the patient is being transported that there is a do not resuscitate order. The individual on the receiving end of this communication should be one who will be responsible for seeing to it that this order is respected while the patient is in his or her department.

The committee considered and rejected proposals to employ a standard identifying symbol affixed either to the patient, to the medical record, or to the bed or stretcher. The basis for this rejection was that it was too dangerous; such symbols might inadvertently be left on the stretcher, for example, when a new patient used it. Similarly rejected was a proposal to write do not resuscitate orders on requisitions for such services as x-rays; the grounds for this rejection were that the requisition tends not to remain in the immediate vicinity of the patient.

NOTE

1.   Members of the Committee on Policy for Do Not Resuscitate Decisions are as follows:

Shirley Blood, R.N., Head Nurse, Clinical Research Center, Yale–New Haven Hospital.

John F. D'Avella, M.D., Fellow, Section of Nephrology, Department of Medicine, Yale University School of Medicine; formerly Chief Medical Resident, Yale–New Haven Hospital.

Constance T. Donovan, R.N., M.S.N., Assistant Professor, Medical-Surgical Nursing Program, Yale School of Nursing, and Clinical Nurse Specialist, Yale–New Haven Hospital.

Thomas P. Duffy, M.D., Associate Professor of Medicine, Yale University School of Medicine.

David C. Duncombe, M.Div., Ph.D., Chaplain, Yale University School of Medicine, and Assistant Professor of Pastoral Theology, Yale Divinity School.

Angela R. Holder, LL.M., Counsel for Medicolegal Affairs, Yale–New Haven Hospital, and Associate Clinical Professor of Pediatrics (Law), Yale University School of Medicine.

Robert J. Levine, M.D. (Chair), Professor of Medicine and Lecturer in Pharmacology, Yale University School of Medicine.

Melvin Lewis, M.B., F.R.C. Psych., D.C.H., Professor of Pediatrics and Psychiatry and Director of Medical Studies, Child Study Center, Yale University School of Medicine.

Kathleen A. Nolan, Yale Medical Student.

Rosalind A. Reed, R.N., Staff Nurse, Medical Intensive Care Unit, Yale–New Haven Hospital.

James A. Talcott, Yale Medical Student.

Deciding to Stop: Physician-Patient Interactions in Oncology

Marianne Prout, M.D.

2

I would like to talk about some of the very pragmatic considerations that I encounter daily as an oncologist. Although I believe that most critical treatment or nontreatment decisions should be made individually among the particular physicians, nurses, patients, and their families, the overriding issues are sensitive and belong in a public forum. We need to expose our thought processes.

When I realize that a patient has failed all therapy that seems reasonable and is likely to afford remission of the disease, that the patient is headed on an inevitable course within an inevitable time, and that nothing I can do will change either the course or the time, I sit down and talk frankly with the patient to ascertain in detail the patient's own desires. I try to find out what matters most to these patients and list their priorities. Patients are often very blunt about their concerns and desires and may express their priorities with statements like, "Number one, I don't want to have any pain; number two, I want to go to my daughter's wedding; number three, I want to die at home," or "I don't want to die in the hospital," or "I don't want my children to see me." It is very important to find out what these priorities are; medical and comfort decisions can then be made around the patient's wishes.

Usually these talks occur spontaneously in the course of a chronic illness, but sometimes I may have to provoke the discussion gently. I try to have a witness present, often a member of the nursing team, and I summarize the patient's priorities on the chart. Throughout the process, I also speak with family, friends, and other medical personnel as opportunities arise. I discuss the patient's desires in very specific terms, frequently detailing conversations and exact dates and time periods during which the patient expressed a certain point of view. I want to assure the family that it was not a transient wish made in a time of pain.

My prevailing guideline, like that of most physicians, is to avoid conflicts. Although many physicians try to avoid conflicts because, they say, they do not want to go to court, I believe that we avoid conflict situations because they are painful for everyone, and the situation is already painful enough. Therefore, I make a concerted effort to have the patient, family, and entire health care team working for the same goals and priorities. I will not pursue a course that offends the philosophy of the family, the nurses, the aides, or anyone else who has contact with the family or the patient.

If there is a conflict, I try to set up discussions and counseling in the hope of resolving it before it mounts. This is important. None of us can handle the burden of what we think is a wrong choice in patient care. If anyone involved comes away with a sense of guilt about the medical decisions made, the result is an unnecessary burden that is very hard to bear.

One of the implications of this procedure is that we often explain to all parties involved in very frank terms exactly what the terminal events might be and how they might be handled. I call this avoiding the Chinese fire-drill syndrome. Those of us in the medical profession know that the typical situation is a long drawn-out chronic disease, followed by an acute event that was not anticipated by the people who are there at the very minute; the people present react instinctively, going through all the routine emergency medical procedures. This endeavor is frequently futile and is disheartening to the patient and family alike.

So, we try to be very blunt. For example, a lot of our families want the patient to die at home. But if the patient is likely to have a fatal hemoptysis, to cough up a large amount of blood and die choking on it, the family members must anticipate that; otherwise, their reaction would be like anyone else's — to call for an ambulance, to seek help. We must therefore give extremely frank details if we want to prevent such a frightening situation, not only for the family's sake, but also for the sake of the health professionals. My nursing crew has become very good at standing and comforting a patient who is having a fatal bleed. That is very tough to do, but unless they have been forewarned, they really cannot handle it.

Fortunately, conflicts seldom arise, and I can often sense ahead of time when one might occur, whether it is within the family or among the staff. If the conflict is between the family and the patient, I try to talk with the family, emphasizing that since I am the patient's physician, my contract with the patient is my first priority. I explain that I will help them in any way that I can, but that first I must do what the patient wishes. I may arrange for counseling for the family. Some of the best counselors are other patients, who may be able to convince the family of the patient's point of view and why, for example, further therapy may not be desirable.

If the conflict persists, a compromise may be worked out. Personally, I do not find it morally offensive to insert an IV in an obtunded patient at the family's request if I know that it is not hurting the patient or prolonging the patient's life. If this helps the family feel more comfortable, then the patient is better off, because a family that is comfortable can more easily stay with the patient until the end. Sometimes we do have to make minor compromises. I certainly would not recommend full resuscitation as a compromise. If that is the conflict, then clearly, outside help is needed.

Turning now to other issues, I want to mention some of my personal opinions. Although this is a very difficult area with immense emotional and moral value conflicts and with life-and-death questions, I believe that with very few exceptions, these questions should be resolved outside the framework of the legal profession and the court system. For the most part, these decisions are sad and emotional, painful and time-consuming, but they are not legally questionable.

I do agree that recent court decisions have given us some very important guidelines, defining the limits within which physicians, nurses, patients, and families can move in evaluating a patient's rights versus the prolongation of life. It is comforting to know that the courts will back us up when we are uncertain about our own moral positions or when we are at the limits of what is standard in society's ethical behavior pattern. But I do not think that physicians should look to the court system to get out of tough cases or tight decisions; by "tight," I do not mean legally ambiguous problems, but decisions that are sorrowful and emotionally painful. This is a burden that physicians have always had to bear.

I also believe that a physician's value system influences the technical decisions that are made. People who work with dying patients need to expand the limits of their own value systems. We need to read carefully the legal decisions in the landmark cases; we need to study the ethical dilemmas regarding terminally ill patients; and we need to contemplate our own motives, emotions, and values. And I would hope that those of us who continue to work in this area will expand our range of values so that patients will not have to choose physicians whose values match theirs, but rather that physicians will be able to move within the range of each patient's values.

BIBLIOGRAPHY

Brown, N. K.; Brown, M. A.; and Thompson, D. Decision making for the terminally ill patient. In *Cancer: the behavioral dimensions*, ed. J. W. Cullen, B. H. Fox, and R. N. Isom. New York: Raven Press, 1976.

Crane, D. *The sanctity of social life: physicians' treatment of critically ill patients*. New York: Russell Sage Foundation, 1975.

Dawson, J. J., and Luce, J. K. Quality of life. *Semin. Oncol.* 2:323–327, 1975.

Donahue, W. T. Maintaining dignity of patients. In *Ethical considerations in long term care*, ed. W. E. Winston and A. J. E. Wilson. St. Petersburg, Fla.: Eckered College Gerontology Center, 1977, pp. 157–170.

Konior, G. S., and Levine, A. S. The fear of dying: how patients and their doctors behave. *Semin. Oncol.* 2:311–316, 1975.

Thomas, L. Death in the open. In *The lives of a cell*. New York: The Viking Press, 1974, pp. 113–116.

Veatch, R. M. *Death, dying, and the biological revolution.* New Haven: Yale University Press, 1976.

Verwoerdt, A. *Communication with the fatally ill.* Springfield, Ill.: Charles C Thomas, 1966.

Nurses and Nontreatment Decisions

Catherine P. Murphy, R.N. Ed.D.

3

Nontreatment decisions are frequently encountered in nursing practice, and they pose especially serious dilemmas for many nurses. Only within the past few days, I have become aware of two particular nontreatment decisions that typify what nurses face in their daily practice. In one instance, a decision not to treat a 21-year-old woman was determined by the allocation of resources, the unavailability of a bed in a bone-marrow transplant center.

In the second instance, a nurse practitioner reported how a patient sought her services for a recently diagnosed problem of "indigestion" that was not responding to the physician's prescribed medication of an antacid. The patient claimed that she had recently undergone numerous tests, including a gastrointestinal series, and that her physician found no abnormality other than a case of indigestion. When the patient had a new series of tests, she was found to have a malignant tumor of the stomach, which must have been present at the time of her first x-ray. The nurse's interpretation of the situation was that, because the patient was elderly, the physician decided not to treat her nor to inform her of her condition. On being told of her condition and counseled about the options available, the woman stated that she very much wanted to live, and she chose to have a gastrectomy. Since then, the woman tolerated the surgery well, and her symptoms have subsided.

Since nurses traditionally have had little or no role in the decision-making process about the care of their patients, they have the dual problem of implementing decisions and facing the consequences of such decisions without having been included in making the decisions. The difficulties that nurses encounter in relation to decisions not to treat a patient fall under three broad categories. The first is when there is a conflict with the physician's decision not to give treatment. The problem may be a conflict of philosophies; the nurse's own value system may differ from the physician's. The conflict may also be between the patient's or the family's expressed wishes and the physician's decision. For example, the patient or family may want treatment, but the physician has decided not to give it, sometimes without even informing the patient or family. But a conflict may also arise if the nurse feels that the physician is not correct in the assessment of the patient's condition, the available options for treatment, or the prognosis of the patient's disease.

The second type of problem for nurses is when no decision has been made as to whether or not to treat a patient—or, if a decision has been made, it has not been communicated to the nursing staff. This difficulty can also occur in unforeseen emergencies, such as a sudden change in a patient's condition. Because physicians are increasingly concerned about liability, decisions like these are sometimes purposefully not communicated publicly, and nurses remain in limbo when trying to decide the type of care the patient should receive.

The third troublesome category comprises "benign neglect" nontreatment decisions, in which physicians decide to withhold treatment but do not write orders or state it anywhere on the patient's records. Instead, what often happens is that nurses may be told to walk slowly to the phone if the patient has a cardiac arrest or not to work so hard at preventing complications such as pneumonia, malnutrition, or skin breakdown.

All these situations pose very serious problems. Even when physicians do write orders for nontreatment, nurses are accountable socially and legally for their own actions. Legal precedent for the administration of drugs and treatment is sufficiently clear. Any nurse who administers a wrong dosage of medication is legally responsible for that action, even though the dosage may have been prescribed by a physician. To my knowledge, there have been few if any court cases where a nurse has been liable for erroneously following a physician's order not to treat a patient, but it is not at all unlikely that such cases might occur in the future. This is especially true in light of the increasing autonomy and accountability of practicing nurses.

A question frequently asked is how nurses feel about nontreatment decisions. In the first place, nurses are members of society, and thus, in many ways, they reflect the values of society in general. Some nurses are avid upholders of the sanctity of life and believe that life should be prolonged at all costs. Others are quick to make utilitarian decisions about the quality of life or the costs versus benefits of caring for seriously ill patients, and they may be in favor of nontreatment decisions in almost all cases.

In one study comparing nurses' attitudes with those of physicians', nurses showed more desire for a change in social customs to allow for some form of negative or passive euthanasia.[1] Eighty-five percent of the nurses surveyed stated that they would practice negative euthanasia if the patient or family had signed such authorization. Sixty-eight percent were uncomfortable when physicians did not practice negative euthanasia in terminally ill patients, whereas only 28 percent were uncomfortable when physicians did practice it.

Let me turn to the role nurses should play in the decision to treat or not treat patients. In the bureaucracy of the hospital, nurses are in a line position; they are accountable to the administrative hierarchy and are paid employees of the institution. In addition, they are also accountable to the physicians. This dual chain of command has severely limited the decision-making role available to them. A range of empirical studies supports the contention that physicians have always been central to the decision-making process, while nurses have been relegated to the role of implementing those decisions. At the same time, however, physicians can avoid patients, thus also avoiding the consequences of their decisions. Nurses, meanwhile, must remain with the patients and their families and must face the consequences of the physicians' decisions day after day. Of late, the situation has become much more complex, with hospital lawyers, administrators, and the courts entering into such decisions. I strongly believe that nurses should play a significant role in decisions to treat or not treat their patients.

Paul Ramsey holds that the ultimate and binding requirement for legitimate participation in the ethical decision-making process for health care providers is in their capacity as caregivers, not as curegivers. For Ramsey, the basis of care becomes the source of our particular moral obligation and the court of final appeal for deciding the features of our practice that make what we do right or wrong.[2] In the course of caring, Ramsey maintains that we have to be concerned with two sorts of questions. First, when we are faced with an ethical dilemma, we must ask which of our actions in the situation takes most care of human life. Second, we must also be concerned about the rules of the game in practice and must ask what rules of practice will render actions that are most careful and respectful of the dignity of all concerned in the situation.

In looking at the first question, clearly the nurse is the member of the health care team who renders the most care to patients. Nurses are responsible for the minute-by-minute care of patients in the course of each day. And patients recognize this; they communicate their fears, desires, and wants to nurses much more readily than they do to other health care professionals. In the study comparing nurses' attitudes with those of physicians, it was found that patients discussed the prolonging or shortening of their lives far more often with nurses than with physicians.[3] In the surgical-specialty services, for example, 35 percent of the nurses reported that they had heard requests from patients for positive euthanasia, while only 3 percent of the physicians had received such requests.

Nurses are also in the best position to assess how patients interact as social beings. They are the ones who observe the psychological state of an ill person in the course of a day and see how the patient interacts with family and friends. From their vantage point and intimate contact with patients, nurses are able to judge how meaningful an existence a critically ill patient has.

I do not wish to negate the role of physicians in making such decisions. They are the experts in diagnosing, treating, and predicting the course of the disease process; their technical and scientific knowledge and expertise are indispensable. However, nurses, more than any other members of the health care team, are in a position to judge the quality of a patient's existence and the meaning of life for that patient. Indeed, many states now formally recognize the value of the nurses' position, and recently updated versions of the Nurse Practice Act state clearly that nurses are concerned with how patients respond and cope with illness. Physicians make diagnoses about a patient's disease process, and nurses make diagnoses about the way the patient is coping with that process.

Decisions to treat or not to treat patients are complex. They incorporate scientific and technical evaluations as well as value judgments about the quality of life. Physicians obviously have the expertise for scientific aspects, while nurses have the expertise for value judgments about the quality of life for a particular patient. Physicians, nurses, social workers, clergy, and other members of the health care team should all be involved in making decisions when they have played a significant role in caring for the patient.

Lest I appear to be fighting a custody battle over who shall make the decisions, let me state that when at all possible, it ought to be the patients themselves who decide whether they should live or die. To quote Bertram and Elsie Bandman, "If there are any moral rights at all, there is at least one prior right founded on justice—the equal right of all persons to be free to decide to live or die."[4]

Some would argue that it is more benevolent to exclude patients from the decision-making process when their very lives conflict with their need for comfort and relief of misery. Much of the discussion on dying these days is concerned with dignified death, or death with dignity. Marvin Kohl tells us that dignity "connotes having reasonable control over the major and significant aspects of one's life, as well as the ofttimes necessary condition of not being treated disrespectfully."[5] He explains further that to have dignity is to have the actual ability to determine and control one's way of life and death rationally and to have this fact acknowledged and respected by others. All human beings have a basic need for dignity and thus a corresponding right to be so treated.

Let me end with another quote from the Bandmans: "No amount of kindness or benevolence can ever justify depriving a person of his right to consent or to refuse to have his life medically terminated."[6] There is no death with dignity if you do not respect the patients' right to be free to decide whether they want to live or die.

REFERENCES

1.   Brown, N. K., et al. How do nurses feel about euthanasia and abortion? *Am. J. Nurs.* 71:1413–1416, 1971.

2.   Ramsey, P. Conceptual foundations for an ethics of medical care: a response. In *Ethics and health policy,* ed. R. M. Veatch and R. Branson. Cambridge, Mass.: Ballinger, 1976, pp. 48–55.

3.   Brown, N. K., et al. How do nurses feel abut euthanasia and abortion? pp. 1413–1416.

4.   Bandman, B., and Bandman, E. Rights, justice, and euthanasia. In *Beneficent euthanasia,* ed. M. Kohl. New York: Prometheus Books, 1975, p. 81.

5.   Kohl, M. Voluntary beneficent euthanasia. In *Beneficent euthanasia,* ed. M. Kohl. New York: Prometheus Books, 1975, p. 133.

6.   Bandman, B., and Bandman, E. Rights, justice, and euthanasia. p. 92.

Legal Limits on the Rights to Refuse Treatment

Leonard H. Glantz, J.D.

4

In preparing this presentation, I reviewed a number of legal cases to see what the limits actually are on the right to refuse treatment. In fact, there are very few cases in which a court has ordered treatment for a patient who was unwilling to undergo that treatment, and that includes all the Jehovah's Witness cases, which people tend to believe epitomize forced treatment. None of the major Jehovah's Witness cases that I reviewed concerns a patient who does not want treatment. What these cases deal with are patients who do not want to consent to blood transfusions, and I emphasize "do not want to consent." Let me give a few examples.

Perhaps the most famous case was in 1964 in Georgetown Hospital, involving a Jehovah's Witness who needed blood in order to survive.[1] She was 25 years old and had a 7-month-old child. Her husband told the judge, who visited the patient at her bedside, that if the transfusion were ordered by the court, responsibility for the transfusion would be the court's and not theirs. The patient agreed that the responsibility would be the judge's and not hers. Thus in this case, while the patient and her husband would not consent to a blood transfusion, they did not oppose it.

A year later, in *United States* v. *George*,[2] a 39-year-old father of four who had lost 60 to 65 percent of his red blood cells refused to consent to a transfusion. According to the court, he had signed a release form and was coherent and rational. When the judge entered his room, the first thing the patient said—before the judge asked him anything—was that he would not agree to the transfusion, but in no way would he resist if the court ordered it. He maintained that if the court ordered the transfusion, it would be the court's will and not his; his conscience would be "clear," and the responsibility for the act would be "upon the court's conscience." The judge explained that he had no power to force the transfusion and that the patient would be free to resist the transfusion by putting his hand over the site where the needle would be injected. Mr. George replied that once the court order was signed, he would in no way resist the transfusion.

These cases are generally referred to as supporting the concept of compelled treatment. Let me compare them to *In re Osborne*,[3] a 1972 case concerning a 34-year-old father of two who was seriously injured and needed blood transfusions. He also was a Jehovah's Witness. When queried by the judge, he expressed the belief that he would be deprived of everlasting life if the judge ordered him to be given a transfusion. The patient said, "It is between me and Jehovah, not the courts. . . . I'm willing to take my chances. My faith is that strong. I wish to live, but with no blood transfusions. Now get that straight!"[4] In this case, no transfusion was ordered.

Thus, we have to distinguish between cases in which people actually refused blood transfusions or treatment and those in which people refused to consent to treatment but were willing to undergo it if the judge consented for them. Judges hear these differences very clearly and deal with them accordingly. There is really no case, with perhaps one exception, in which the court ordered a screaming, kicking, competent person to be restrained and given a transfusion. There is also no case, with one possible recent exception, in which a competent person has been required to undergo any procedure more invasive than a blood transfusion; I will return to that exception later.

I think it is fair to say that today, most, if not all, courts start out with the proposition that a competent adult has the right to refuse treatment even if such nontreatment leads to the person's death. Two occurrences have made this true. One is the increasing acceptance by the courts of the doctrine of informed consent. The second has to do with *Roe* v. *Wade*,[5] the 1973 United States Supreme Court abortion case that explicated the concept of the constitutional right to privacy. Courts that have dealt with the right to nontreatment since 1973 have discussed the issue of the right to privacy and have adopted it.[6] They have said, for the most part, that the right to privacy includes the right to refuse treatment. Thus, in discussing and analyzing this type of case, we need to differentiate between pre-1973 cases and post-1973 cases because, on the whole, the pre-1973 cases do not discuss that constitutional right. For example, the New Jersey Supreme Court in 1971, in the *Heston*[7] case, said that there is no constitutional right to die, but in 1976, in the *Quinlan*[8] case, the same court held that the constitutional right to privacy encompasses the right to refuse treatment. Conceptually, 1973 serves as a boundary.

No court, though, has said that the right to refuse treatment is absolute. There are state interests that permit a state to abridge the right to refuse treatment. These state interests, as defined by the courts, are (1) the preservation of life, (2) the protection of innocent third parties, (3) the prevention of suicide, and (4) the maintaining of the ethical integrity of the medical profession. But there is another interest, which I would call "4A," that is found in some courts and most specifically in New Jersey: the "right" of physicians to administer medical treatment according to their best judgment.

The easiest state interest to discuss is the prevention of suicide. Although the *Heston* court in New Jersey in 1971 said that refusing lifesaving treatment is tantamount to suicide, all other recent courts have said that it is not, including the *Quinlan* court. To commit suicide, according to the law, a person has to have specific intent to die and the individual must purposely set in motion the death-producing agent.[9] In most of the cases that we are talking about, the first criterion is missing; these individuals do not want to die, but they do not want to be treated and would accept death as a consequence of nontreatment. The second condition is also absent; the individuals do not set the death-producing agent into motion, since they have not produced their illnesses or conditions.

Regarding the state interest in the preservation of life, the courts agree that preserving human life must be balanced against the traumatic cost of saving that life. In *Quinlan*, the New Jersey court stated that as the degree of bodily invasion increases and the prognosis dims, the state's interest in preserving that life decreases.[10] More recently, courts in both New Jersey[11] and Massachusetts[12] have agreed that the focus can be on the nature of the invasion to the patient and that the idea of prognosis can be put aside for the most part. Thus, both courts refused to order amputations of the legs of individuals who did not want such treatment in situations where nontreatment might lead to death. These decisions were based on the level of bodily invasion and not on the possibly poor prognosis. I believe that part of their reasoning is that, in some senses, a "good" prognosis involves a value judgment. To say that being in a wheelchair or being bedridden is a good or a poor prognosis is a personal, subjective decision, and that is the sort of choice that only individual patients are capable of making under the doctrine of informed consent.

In terms of the state's interest in the preservation of human life, one court observed that the "notion that an individual exists for the good of the state is, of course, quite antithetical to our fundamental thesis that the role of the state is to ensure a maximum of individual freedom of choice and conduct."[13] Courts are beginning to question precisely what the state interest is in preserving the life of someone who does not want to be treated. Certainly, the state has a strong interest in preserving life that might be irrationally taken, and certainly, it has a very strong interest in preserving life that might be involuntarily taken. But to what extent does the state have an interest in preserving the life of a competent person who does not want treatment when that nontreatment will lead to death?

Another state interest is that of maintaining the ethical integrity of the medical profession. In *Saikewicz*, the court found that medical ethics permitted the refusal of treatment by a competent patient. Physicians are not required by medical ethics to treat competent patients against their will, however; at least, I have seen no indications that physicians are supposed to hold down patients and treat them against their will, especially with invasive treatments. A second point involving the maintenance of the ethical integrity of the medical profession is that courts will not force doctors to administer poor care, that is, to do things they believe to be bad medical practice. So if a Jehovah's Witness refuses blood, courts do not insist that a surgeon operate on that person in the absence of blood.

The right of physicians to administer medical treatment according to their best judgment, however, is a state interest that had not occurred to me before reading these cases. This interest usually arises when a court says, for example, that a patient is victimizing the health care providers by not allowing them to practice their profession, thus placing them in an awkward situation.[14] This certainly causes a bind for health care providers and presents difficult ethical and personal problems. But I think it is nonsense to say that health care providers have a legal right to practice their profession on a specific patient. I do not believe there is any source for such a right. If such a right did exist, the concepts of informed consent and personal autonomy would be totally negated. The concept of informed consent means that although physicians understand the risks and benefits of a suggested procedure, only the patients themselves can weigh those risks and benefits against their own subjective needs and fears and finally decide whether to undergo the treatment.

Perhaps the most difficult and most important counterbalancing right of the state is its interest in protecting innocent third parties, particularly minors. This very difficult issue comes up repeatedly in many of the cases I discussed. Some patients refusing treatment had minor children, and the courts drew attention to that as being an important interest.

Courts talk about protecting children in two ways. One is that the child might become a ward of the state. Some courts say that the child's material well-being may be sacrificed or the child may suffer psychological harm if the parent is allowed to die. The first concern, that of the child becoming a ward of the state, seems not to recognize that most children have two parents and thus would not become orphans if one parent dies. In the *Osborne* case, the court actually examined the second concern very factually, looking at the family and asking about the children's material needs. The testimony showed that all the children's material needs would be taken care of since the family business would continue even if the father died. A close extended family was also available to support the children in a variety of ways.

Although I can understand why courts for very human

reasons consider these factors, such consideration raises a number of problems. One is the specter of being too poor to refuse treatment; that is, an individual can refuse treatment if the family is well taken care of but must undergo treatment if the children are dependent on the refusing party's salary. I suppose someone could get life insurance to insure the right to refuse treatment, but that seems an odd way to solve the problem. If financial impact on the family is going to be used as a criterion for such decisions, then to be fair, we should look equally at the possible negative consequences of treatment if that treatment would produce a financial burden. We might then have to suggest nontreatment if the family would suffer financially if the treatment were rendered. If we use financial considerations, we have to use them in both directions. Wealth as a criterion causes serious problems, especially if it is being used to determine whether or not an individual can exercise a constitutional right to privacy. It makes me very uncomfortable, and I believe an individual's wealth should not determine that person's right to refuse treatment.

Psychological harm to children is difficult to assess in any individual case. We would have to look at the developmental issues related to the specific children. If the child is a newborn, perhaps the psychological harm would be less than if the child were a bit older. It is difficult—if not impossible—to determine the severity of the harm, to measure psychological harm in any particular instance. What if the parent and child do not get along? What if the parent is a child abuser? Would these conditions argue in favor of a person exercising a right to nontreatment? Do bad parents have a greater right to refuse treatment than good parents?

But even if we could assess psychological or material harm, we face the question of whether it is fair or desirable to treat one person for the benefit of another, regardless of whether the "benefit" is for a child, a spouse, or an elderly parent. If the answer is yes, we raise additional problems. For example, if a parent can be compelled to undergo a medical procedure for the well-being of a child, can a parent who would be a compatible donor be forced to donate a kidney to a child who needs one? As soon as we start talking about treating one person for the benefit of another, we have to be willing to answer this type of question.

The case that is perhaps most often quoted for the proposition that one can treat a parent in order to save a child also took place in New Jersey, in 1964. The case, *Raleigh Fitkin-Paul Morgan Memorial Hospital* v. *Anderson*,[15] involved a pregnant Jehovah's Witness who required a transfusion to save the life of her fetus. Here we have a situation in which the benefit is very direct. The court decided that the state had an interest in protecting the life of the "unborn child" and ordered that the woman be given a blood transfusion to protect that life. The case is widely quoted, but I question whether it is good law anymore. It is a pre-1973 case, and since then, *Roe* v. *Wade* has said that a woman can choose to have an abortion. After *Roe* v. *Wade*, *Raleigh* can still have force only if it is argued that a pregnant woman is required to have an abortion in order to refuse treatment or that she is now entitled to take action that will lead to the death of the fetus but cannot direct inaction that would lead to a similar death. Because of the outright silliness of these interpretations, I would say that this 1964 case is no longer good law; the courts should stop relying on this case and should reexamine the cases that depended on it in the past.

I also want to mention the final resolution of this case. The defendant, Ms. Anderson, left the hospital against medical advice, without being given a transfusion, and the court never said and never intimated that she could be forceably returned to the hospital in order to save the fetus or herself.

Earlier, I mentioned an exceptional recent case. This is the case of *Hall* v. *Myers*.[16] Mr. Hall is the Commissioner of Corrections in Massachusetts, and Mr. Myers is a 25-year-old inmate at one of the state's correctional institutions. Mr. Myers has kidney disease requiring dialysis, and he has refused the dialysis. At some point, he withdrew his consent for dialysis, basically for political reasons. He said that the dialysis made him weak, that he did not believe that he could protect himself adequately at that particular prison, and that he wished to be transferred to a less secure facility. When his request for transfer was denied, he withdrew his consent to the dialysis.

The commissioner obtained an injunction to require the inmate to undergo kidney dialysis. In court, physicians testified that it would be possible to restrain Mr. Myers in order to make him undergo dialysis; other testimony refers to the use of handcuffs and manacles and to the fact that strong correctional officers had the ability to hold him down. It was suggested that as long as they could restrain him three times a week, they would be able to treat him adequately. The testimony also pointed out that his treatments were accompanied by nausea, headaches, and exhaustion. The court said that Mr. Myers was competent, that he had no wish to die, but that he did not wish to be treated. The commissioner maintained that permitting Mr. Myers to refuse treatment would be contrary to proper prison administration. Actually, this is a combination of two types of cases, a prisoner's rights case and a patient's rights case.

What the court decided—and this refers back to what we have been saying about people making value judgments for other people—is that dialysis is not really a very intrusive treatment. The court stated that this sort of procedure is certainly less painful than chemotherapy, the proposed treatment in the *Saikewicz* case, and therefore cannot be considered especially intrusive. The court also found no problem with the use of physical restraint, because the patient was already a prisoner. According to the court, it was up to the commissioner to determine where the prisoner's time was to be spent, and it probably would not make much difference to the prisoner whether he spent his time in a prison cell or on a dialysis machine. In fact, the court added, some prisoners would be happy to be let out of prison in exchange for dialysis. The court said that 15 hours a week on a machine rather than in prison "cannot be deemed particularly offensive."

In summary, there are two significant aspects in this decision. One is that the court compelled treatment because of its belief that dialysis under restraint is a relatively unobtrusive procedure. The second is that physical restraint was found to be permissible, and even more so because Mr. Myers is a prisoner. The court went on to admit that its decision is contrary to the weight of authority in all other jurisdictions and that it strongly believes that competent patients generally have the right to refuse lifesaving treatment. The judge said that none of the decisions in Massachusetts compels the outcome the court came to, although they do support this outcome. The judge then added that the decision requiring treatment made him more comfortable and that if he is to make a mistake, he intends to err on the side of life. Furthermore, the judge reported this case to the Supreme Judicial Court, where it is still pending.

To me, this case constitutes an outrageous intrusion on the

physical privacy of a competent person, and it demonstrates the problems involved in compulsory treatment, especially treatment that is more invasive than a blood transfusion. I believe that this case is an aberration and that the appellate court will reverse it; I certainly hope it does.

Until very recently, with the advent of "natural death" legislation, the entire corpus of law regarding nontreatment has been written by judges. When judges are asked to permit people to make decisions that may lead to their death, they are put in a very difficult position. Neither their training nor their experiences have prepared them to make life-or-death decisions. By permitting the use of, at times, relatively unintrusive treatments, judges can apparently save the life of an unwilling patient. Emotionally, there are very powerful reasons why a judge, given the choice, would order such a treatment. We can only hope that judges will continue their practice of dispassionately balancing the rights of individuals against the interests of the state and contemplating the long-range effect of their decisions. In the past, judges have been mostly concerned with defining the rights of the individual. It now seems clear that individuals do indeed have the right to refuse treatment. Future litigation should focus on defining the state's interest in abridging the right of the individual to decide whether or not to undergo treatment.

As I hope I have demonstrated, the interests of the state are not so powerful nor so logically based as they appear to be. If judges continue to examine these cases as they have recently, we can feel safe that the averred interests of the state will not overwhelm individual freedom.

NOTES

1.   *Applications of the President and Directors of Georgetown College*, 331 F.2d 1000 (D.C. Cir. 1964).

2.   *United States* v. *George*, 239 F. Supp. 752 (Conn. 1965).

3.   *In re Osborne*, 294 A.2d 372 (D.C. Ct. of Appeals 1972).

4.   *Id* at 374.

5.   *Roe* v. *Wade*, 410 U.S. 113 (1973).

6.   See, e.g., *In the Matter of Karen Quinlan*, 70 N.J. 10, 355 A.2d 647 at 662–664 (1976).

7.   *John F. Kennedy Memorial Hospital* v. *Heston*, 58 N.J. 576, 279 A.2d 670 (1971).

8.   *Supra* note 6.

9.   Byrn, R. M. Compulsory life saving treatment for the competent adult. *Fordham Law Review* 44:16–24, 1975.

10.   *Supra* note 6 at 355 A.2d at 664.

11.   *In the Matter of Quackenbush*, 156 N.J. Super. 282, 383 A.2d 785 (Morris County Ct. 1978).

12.   *Lane* v. *Candura* 376 N.E.2d 1232 (Mass. App. 1978).

13.   *Supra* note 3 at 375 n.5.

14.   *Supra* note 7 at 279 A.2d at 673–674.

15.   *Raleigh Fitkin-Paul Morgan Memorial Hospital* v. *Anderson*, 42 N.J. 421, 201 A.2d 537 (1964).

16.   *Hall* v. *Myers*, No. 32245 (Mass. Suffolk Sup. Ct., Jan. 8. 1979). After this paper was written, the Supreme Court upheld the lower court and decided that the prisoner could be forced to undergo hemodialysis. See *Commissioner of Corrections* v. *Myers*, 399 N.E.2d 452 (Mass. 1979).

Discussion

Harvey W. Freishtat, J.D., Moderator

5

Mr. Freishtat: As moderator, I have the privilege of asking the first question, which I shall address to Dr. Levine. When you were talking about Yale's authorization scheme, it sounded as if you were somehow differentiating that scheme from what we familiarly call informed consent. From what I have heard, though, it seems in keeping with informed consent, in that the physician presents the patient with the facts and then gives a recommendation. But I take it that in your mind, there is a difference, that there is more of a value judgment seeping into the exchange. Would you elaborate?

Dr. Levine: I'm not sure that there is a fundamental difference between what I'm calling authorization and informed consent. When I talk about authorization, I am referring to a situation in which there really are no reasonable alternatives. You cannot walk up to patients who are on the verge of death and ask them whether they want to be cured. It would be brutal to approach the family and say, "Your relative is comatose; we see no possibility of reversing anything. We can continue to resuscitate for a long time, but the decision is strictly up to you."

Basically, we convey the same sort of information, but in a

different way. Perhaps we say that it is possible to resuscitate and to maintain respiration and nutrition, but we recommend against it because there seems to be no likelihood that the patient will ever experience anything again or be able to communicate the experience. We do not necessarily put the choice to the person; rather, we ask authorization to assume the total burden. It is one thing for a family to say, "I chose to turn off grandma's respirator," and it is quite another thing to say, "I went along with the doctor's recommendation that it was time to turn off grandma's respirator."

It is easy to charge that this is a return to the old paternalistic, doctor-knows-best situation. I want to emphasize that I'm talking in a context where the relationship between the doctor and patient has been defined as early as possible in an effort to find out how the patient would want things to be handled.

I am not as sanguine as Dr. Prout is about the capability of physicians generally to expand the range of values that they can cope with. I think it is possible for all of us, through our experience, studies, and conversations, to become aware of a larger range of values than those we grew up with, but I believe that we all tend to have our own sets of values that influence the way we see things, even when we try to be objective. To the extent that we can be aware of ourselves and to the extent that our values may become relevant to a particular doctor-patient relationship, it is very important to clarify early in the relationship those values that influence the physician. Perhaps the highest order of informed consent is to inform the patient of those values.

The fundamental ethical basis for informed consent is to show respect for a person as a self-determining agent. One of the ways we can show respect for a person who happens now to be in the role of patient is to say, "You're in charge; you have the authority to make decisions. One of your decisions is to delegate decision-making authority. You also have the authority not to receive any more information than you want; you can delegate the authority to someone else."

Mr. Freishtat: Let me ask Prof. Glantz if, from that description, you see inconsistencies between the authorization dialogue and the basic requirements of informed consent.

Prof. Glantz: I need to begin with a question for Dr. Levine. With the authorization scheme, I believe you're often talking about it in terms of the family; is that right?

Dr. Levine: Most commonly, such talks are with the family because these decisions have to be worked out very near the time that a do not resuscitate order might have been implemented. It is much better, of course, from the perspectives of both the doctor and the patient, if someone has talked with the patient about such things a couple of months earlier.

Prof. Glantz: Ideally, what the physician is doing is putting forward the patient's best interest, as the patient had discussed previously with the physician, and enforcing what the patient had wanted in the past. The authorization scheme, as described here, seems to be one of helping the family come to grips with a decision that ideally the patient and the physician have made together. I do not see that as conflicting with informed consent. Another thing I hear, which is also said about informed consent, is that not everything that a physician has the power to do has to be disclosed. But I believe that the point Dr. Levine is making is that, by this time, the physicians have done all that they can do and there is no alternative to be disclosed. I don't see a conflict.

Dr. Levine: There have been several significant cases that have established the law of informed consent, such as *Cobbs* v. *Grant* and *Canterbury*. I see those cases as setting standards for resolving differences of opinion between doctors and patients, and I think that they, like so many malpractice cases, have to do with failures in the medical system. I do not believe that they should guide us in our ordinary practice of medicine; that would make the whole thing an adversary proceeding. Taking guidance from these cases, which would require us not only to inform everybody fully up to the minimum of the reasonable patient standard, but also to document the fact that we have done so on a signed consent form, would really make us work in an adversary environment.

Most doctor-patient relationships are not discussed in the courtroom. Learning how to practice medicine from studying malpractice cases is akin to learning how to run a marriage counseling service by studying cases that go to divorce court; it tells you what not to do. I don't think we can draw much guidance by examining the failures, usually the grotesque anomalies of the medical practice situation. When informed consent is interpreted as requiring a signed consent form, the only purpose is to defend the doctor against the patient, not to protect the patient's interests.

Dr. Michael Liepman (Departments of Family Practice and Psychiatry, University of Michigan, Ann Arbor): Could someone address, from the legal perspective and from the perspective of good medical care, some of the difficult issues of families of dying competent individuals, especially when an apparent conflict of interest exists between the patient and the family. For example, how do we cope with a situation in which the patient wants to die at home but the family does not want that, or a terminal patient wants extraordinary life-prolonging measures while the family cannot afford the financial drain? How about the person who does not want the family to know of the terminal nature of the illness, yet the family needs to know in order to plan?

Dr. Prout: Those certainly are some of the problems that we run into. The patient wants to die at home, and the family can't cope and is falling apart. How we handle that depends somewhat on what kinds of options we have. Where I work, we are very lucky in having lots of options. We can get outsiders—physicians, nurses, and homemakers—brought into the home so that the family can take a break; at times, we have been able to do that for 24-hour stretches. What we try to determine is whether the family is exhausted and needs a break or whether it is really a no-go situation. We can't tell that in the outpatient clinic, so we get somebody to visit the home. If it's a badly needed vacation, we get whatever coverage is necessary, whether it's a brief hospitalization or help in the home. We give the family a chance to regroup; we also provide counseling in the meantime. If the issue cannot be settled this way, we're left with the inherent problem of patient rights versus family rights. If the family absolutely abandons the patient, there is nothing we can do except to hope that counseling can provide reconciliation.

Regarding patients who want terminal heroic events, I'm afraid that isn't part of my philosophy. I disagree with Dr. Levine; I think that you really can recognize where your values stop and where the patient's begin. Even if a patient's wishes are outside your range, you can go along, as long as you don't think it unconscionable. I believe that patients who want everything done have the right to have everything done. Fortunately, in my system, I am always able to deliver what the patient wants.

What do we do when a patient doesn't want the family to know? That doesn't trouble me so much, although I would want to know the reason. What bothers me more is the family that doesn't want the patient to know, which I think is more common. You have to look at who is trying to protect whom from what and see whether it looks reasonable.

Mr. Freishtat: Dr. Prout, your examples assume competent patients. Would anything you have just said depend on the degree to which the patient is competent? Obviously, in the law, someone is either competent or incompetent, but in medicine, there are myriad shades of gray.

Dr. Prout: Whereas to a lawyer someone is competent or incompetent, when it comes to clinical practice, especially as patients approach the terminal stage, they are almost always "none of the above." It seems that every time I am in a tight spot, I get one of these none-of-the-above arrangements; I can't get anyone to declare a patient incompetent, but neither will anyone declare the patient competent. This is a case where we slug it through and do our best. We could go to court, but I don't think that is reasonable. If a patient has not been declared incompetent, and if you have tried to get such a declaration, then you have to presume that the patient is still in the driver's seat, even though you may not agree with how the driving is done. The majority of cases are in this gray zone; it drives us clinicians crazy, but I accept that as a burden.

Mr. Freishtat: I want to point out that two particular cases concerning the right to refuse treatment were resolved recently by the courts, one in Massachusetts in the *Lane* v. *Candura* case and the other in the *Quackenbush* case in New Jersey. Both cases involved people who had a difference of opinion regarding competence in the medical sense, rather than in the legal sense; both times, the courts erred on the side of competence, upholding the right to refuse treatment.

Mr. Richard Roelofs (Fellow in Bioethics, Montefiore Hospital and Medical Center, Bronx): I'd like to comment on Prof. Glantz's discussion of Jehovah's Witnesses. I believe that there is something a little disreputable about the argument that it is okay to force Jehovah's Witnesses to receive blood transfusions on the grounds that, so long as it is done against their will, no religious guilt will result. It is like saying, "You can do this to me, doc, so long as you do it against my will." This sounds like giving consent to something that is at the same time unconsenting. Morally, I find that disreputable.

Let me also talk about a related case. On Friday the 13th of April, a judge in the Bronx handed down a decision to have a guardian appointed for a person who was 20 years old, which is two years above the age of consent in New York, so that a transfusion could be done on her. She was a Jehovah's Witness and, over the course of her lengthy hospitalization, had repeatedly persisted in refusing to accept a tranfusion. During an *ex parte* proceeding, the woman's father, who had not been part of the family picture for many years, requested the judge to issue an order appointing a hospital administrator as a guardian for the purpose of doing whatever was medically necessary. And medically, transfusion was vital.

My question now is twofold. The hospital wanted to uphold the patient's right to refuse the transfusion but was forced to do the transfusion. Because it was an *ex parte* proceeding, the hospital's lawyers were not allowed to be present to argue against the order. Is there any legal defense against that kind of proceeding? Also, must we anticipate this type of thing happening more often? Perhaps because of Jonestown, the Reverend Moon, or whatever, judges may become readier to hear parents assert their rights to take charge of an adult child's life to protect that adult child against the consequences of religious foolishness or overzealous commitment.

Prof. Glantz: My quick answer is that the defense has to find a good judge. I am not familiar with any case in which a court has told a physician that the physician must give a transfusion to somebody, that is, must go to the bedside and stick a needle in a person's arm. The way it usually works is that a physician will explain that a procedure is medically necessary and ask for authorization to do it even in the absence of the patient's consent. To defend against the instance you raised, I would say that the physician who was charged with the care should come to court and say, "I'm not going to do it. There is no precedent for making a physician do this sort of thing. If you make me do it, I won't be this person's physician anymore." The physician-patient contract is a voluntary one, and it can be broken.

In the case you presented, some facts are not clear. Guardians are not involuntarily appointed, so the hospital administrator must have been willing to become a guardian. The best protection for the rights of individuals comes from the people who work in hospitals, so, if the administrator was appointed guardian, the administrator had some part in it.

Concerning whether the courts will interfere more in the future, let's not talk about cultists and people kidnapping their children. The courts seem to be beginning to say that the fact that someone is a Jehovah's witness probably doesn't make any difference. First amendment and religious questions have pretty much been resolved for the most part. Now the question is whether a competent adult, for whatever reasons, including being a Jehovah's Witness, can decide not to receive care. Thus, I believe that the religious aspects of the question will probably decrease in importance rather than increase. Why the court made that decision for the 20-year old, I don't know. Nor do I know who the petitioners were or why the father came out of nowhere or what the mental state of the person was, so it's difficult to know from the facts that you presented exactly what happened.

As far as Jehovah's Witnesses saying that somebody can do it as long as it is done against their will, I think that you have to ask, what does it mean to do something against somebody's will? What these Jehovah's Witnesses are saying is, "It's not against my will for you to do it, but I won't ask affirmatively for it. I won't ask you to do it, but I will passively accept it." There seems to be a difference between going after something and passively accepting it, and that's the distinction that Jehovah's Witnesses are making in these cases.

Dr. Levine: Let me elaborate a bit. Some years ago, I found that a lot of Jehovah's Witness parents were refusing transfusions, although we could get a court order over the phone opposing their apparent will. I was particularly concerned about the type of case Prof. Glantz presented, in which the patient said he would be eternally damned if he were given a transfusion. I decided to talk to an elder in the Jehovah's Witness Church in New Haven. I asked how the Church deals with a child who receives a blood transfusion by a court order — whether the child is seen as stained, whether the child is excluded, or whether the child will really be damned. His position is that this is a child who has been injured by society; the child is welcomed back in the Church and provided with special care and attention to show that although the child has been assaulted, it is still a good child and a member of the community. His remarks made me feel much better about opposing the apparent will of parents.

Prof. Glantz: I should add that I was talking about competent Jehovah's Witnesses and not about children. Also, while I do not believe that Jehovah's Witnesses and other competent people will be forced to be treated, I do think that their children will be. That should not be surprising. Such children are considered to be mistreated by their parents for religious reasons, and thus they will continue to receive blood transfusions.

Mr. Freishtat: I suspect that there is a difference between decisions rendered by lower courts on the spot in an emergency and those that are made later, sometimes years afterward, when cases wind their way through the appellate courts. While there may indeed be very few if any reported cases of required treatment of competent Jehovah's Witnesses without some mitigating circumstances, I have a feeling that a lot is going on in the superior courts. Judges are human, and whenever they are in doubt, they err on the side of life. If they are wrong, the appellate court will correct them, long after the transfusion has been administered.

Dr. Lothar Gidro-Frank (Psychiatrist, Columbia Presbyterian Hospital, New York): I would like to ask whether Dr. Levine has been able to change the committee system of treating patients. We have the same problem, with both clinic and private patients. At a recent conference, the question arose as to who the patient's doctor was. Nobody knew. Someone finally spoke up and suggested that, of course, the patient had a doctor: Dr. Medicaid. Have you been able to change that system?

Dr. Levine: I can't document any change. The policy I described is still in the proposal state; we are supposed to take final action on it next month. Even though it is only a proposed policy, a fair number of people at Yale–New Haven Hospital are using it. We have suggested that whenever any member of the health care team is unsure of who is in charge, who the responsible physician is, that person should ask the house officer. If the house officer doesn't know, it is up to the chief resident to identify the doctor in charge. Sometimes this involves a couple of phone calls, frequently to the department chairman, but the question must be resolved.

What often happens is that a patient is admitted to the hospital under the order of, say, a primary care physician and later transferred to the intensive care unit; by this time, four or five subspecialty consultants may be involved and the primary care physician, who may have formally or informally referred the patient to one of those consultants, has faded out of the picture. It may not be clear from the record which consultant got the referral. Thus, various consultants start writing orders that may not be compatible with one another. We activate this system as soon as somebody sees something like that going on. We have at least identified whom to ask to find out.

Dr. Gidro-Frank: I understand your problem, and you have tried to answer the question. But you gave only a formal answer. I have a friend in the hospital with a malignancy, and we talk a lot about her illness and her treatment. When I asked her who her doctor was, she replied, "I don't have a doctor. I have a committee taking care of me." I then said, "What about the guy whose name is on the door?" And she said, "He is least of all my doctor. I can't stand him. Look at what he's doing." You have to get to the point where doctors willingly assume the responsibility to be a patient's doctor. It is not enough to call up and have a resident find out who is in charge; you have to have someone accept the mantle.

Dr. Levine: Among the people we have identified who should ask for identification of the doctor in charge is the patient. I also recognize the difference between form and substance. We have attempted to create a policy that makes the responsible physician aware of what obligations go along with the job description. I'm sure there are some people who won't meet their obligations, but we are trying to promote an awareness of this need, and we're hoping that people will increasingly take on the full responsibility of being the physician in charge. I have no documentation that it is happening, but I have hopes.

Dr. Prout: Often, what a patient really wants to know is who is philosophically in charge, and that may not be the person who is medically in charge. For example, in an intensive care unit, the technical subspecialist who may be doing most of the work may not be the person whom the patient regards as philosophically in charge. Will your system identify the medical or the philosophical person in charge?

Dr. Levine: I guess I don't know exactly what it means to be philosophically in charge, but the responsible physician is the one who is supposed to be aware of all the values and technical judgments that are at stake and competing for attention in the decision-making process. Unlike the cardiologist or oncologist, for example, the responsible physician has examined more than the heart or the bone marrow. I'm not impugning subspecialists, but if your main view of a patient is through the bone marrow, you may not be aware that something is going on in the lungs that will render your recommendations unacceptable. The responsible physician should be aware of all the relevant information from all people who have anything important to say about the care of and the interactions with the patient. If the responsible physician doesn't want that responsibility, then it's a good time to find another one.

Mr. Freishtat: Let's call this person who is philosophically in charge a PIC. What if the PIC and the physician in charge happen to be different people? Let's say that the PIC is a nurse, as Prof. Murphy has suggested is often the case. How does the nurse, who is not number one on the medical team but perhaps a better representative of the patient's interests, handle that kind of situation? How formal does the dialogue become?

Prof. Murphy: This situation results in agonizing kinds of decisions. From time to time, I hear of instances where nurses actually take it on themselves to act in the best interests of the patient or the family. A student in my ethics class recently told me about a case involving a premature infant who had all kinds of severe problems right from the start, who was treated with horrendous, extraordinary lifesaving measures. The family was adamant that these measures not be continued, and the child was obviously suffering. One nurse, the so-called primary nurse, the nurse philosophically in charge of that child, took final responsibility herself. When the child arrested, she picked the child up, cuddled it, and waited for it to die without calling the physician. The physician later told her that she was wrong. These instances do occur.

Mr. Freishtat: Should that kind of disagreement between a nurse and a physician be reflected in the patient's chart?

Prof. Murphy: I would recommend it, but it is probably unlikely.

Dr. Levine: Once you agree to become a member of the team, the ordinary rules of responding to what you perceive as your duties, obligations, and prerogatives begin to change. What you said earlier, Prof. Murphy, about the communication problems between nurses and physicians is quite appropriate. What I would like to do is address these things head on. If our recommended policy becomes effective, people have to follow it. I want to emphasize that people with all sorts of job descriptions are on these teams. Whenever any member of the team believes that an important decision has to be made regarding the management of a patient, that member should approach the house officer or the responsible physician and say so. At that point, the house officer or responsible physician agrees to discuss the change, and this is written in the progress notes. What is written is the fact that a management decision about a patient needs to be made, the sorts of decisions involved, and even the time and place where such discussion will take place. In that way, all the people who may have something important to say about it are alerted that they should show up or at least put in their information.

   I am not talking about a hospital ethics committee or a prognosis committee, such as New Jersey has. I'm talking about a little ad hoc group that constructs itself as a committee of people who are truly interested in a particular case. They can get together and provide their input, but once decisions are made, we believe that the team should work together. We do have a bit of an appeals process, but I do not think it is good for someone unilaterally to depart from what the team has agreed to do. It's similar to football—if the wide receiver decides to run to the left instead of the right, the receiver may be wide open, but the ball is going to go to the wrong place.

Prof. Murphy: I would agree with you if the decision really is made by a team, but all too often, it is not a team decision and there is a problem in communication.

Dr. Prout: I have trouble with the team concept. Patients find it so hard to relate to even one professional, especially physicians and sometimes even nurses, that I think it would be even more difficult to relate to a team. Are you saying that a team handles the decision, but there is one person identified who relates to the patient?

Dr. Levine: Obviously, we can't constrain people from talking with one another, but we usually try to identify the team member who seems best capable of talking with a particular patient; this person will be the spokesperson for the team. We say that this person, in relation to this patient, is in charge of discussing things that the team feels need to be discussed. Ideally, that person most often would be the responsible physician. We have seen various situations and heard conversations where the responsible physician, recognizing an inability in this regard, explicitly delegated the authority to another person on the team. Thus, quite a variety of people could actually be handling these discussions.

Now, we're not telling everybody to keep their mouths shut until everyone has the story straight. What we're saying is that these people are talking as individual human beings who happen to be health professionals, but when the discussion involves something like a request for authorization of a management plan, the team must be sure it has gotten together first and considered all the information available.

Dr. Donald Fayh (Coordinator of Medical Affairs, Western Massachusetts Hospital, Westfield, Mass.): I see doctors, nurses, and lawyers on the panel, but I do not see any clinical pastoral counselors. Yet I think they frequently have the best contact with the patient and in conferences can offer solutions that otherwise could not be obtained.

Dr. Levine: I thought that was clear from my remarks. Certainly these people are members of the team, and I do agree with you.

Mr. Howard Telson (Student, Yale University School of Medicine, New Haven, Conn.): One issue that hasn't been addressed yet is what to do when patients don't want any more information or don't want to be involved in the decisions. That question relates back to Dr. Levine's comment about a family being able to say that the doctor recommended that the plug be pulled, rather than it being the family who pulled the plug. It also relates to the Jehovah's Witness cases, where the law says that the patient didn't really refuse treatment. Informed consent implies not only that you give the patient an option, but that the patient is ultimately the one responsible for making the decision. Are we willing to extend that concept such that the patient must be responsible for making the decision, whether or not the patient wants to? Unless the patient is primarily responsible and is given and accepts both the right and the responsibility to make decisions, we are being paternalistic; we are allowing patients a certain amount of freedom, but once they refuse it, the professional takes over. It seems as if lawyers, courts, doctors, and everyone else are assuming roles as professionals, knowing more and having more responsibility than patients. So, my basic question is, are we willing to give patients the responsibility to make decisions, regardless of whether they want it?

Prof. Glantz: That's a good question. When we think of informed consent, we think of it as a right, which, like other rights, can be waived; the decision can be given to somebody else. I am not particularly disturbed by the idea of letting health care providers make certain decisions for others. I think it's different from walking into a bank and saying, "I'm thinking of buying a house. You decide whether I should buy it and what sort of mortgage I should get. Don't consult me at all; just send me the papers." People would find that pretty unusual. However, we're not disturbed when somebody says, "Look, doctor, don't tell me about these risks and benefits. I'm really worried about this operation, but if you think it's okay, then do it for me." The issue of individual responsibility is an important one, and we are willing to say that people can consent to someone else acting paternalistically toward them. That is how I would conceptualize your point. It doesn't particularly bother me. On the other hand, your argument that people should be responsible for themselves is very powerful. It's really a personal value.

Dr. Levine: I think Mr. Telson's question is a very good one, and I would like Prof. Glantz's opinion on an extension of it. If a patient demands to be treated without being fully informed, should we document that on the consent form and have the patient sign it, in the interest of protecting the physician?

Prof. Glantz: You pointed out yourself that the main purpose of documentation is to protect physicians and hospitals against suits, so if I were advising hospitals, I would say yes. Whether or not you let the patient decide is up to you, in terms of its validity, but certainly you should put that in the record.

(Speaker unidentified): I'd like to ask Prof. Glantz about the legal status of living wills. As a nurse, I've seen many patients who I know would prefer not to be treated in an extraordinary manner.

Prof. Glantz: A number of states have statutes dealing with the legal status of living wills. Some states require health professionals to carry out the patient's wishes as stated in a living will. Other states permit health professionals to rely on such documents in making nontreatment decisions but do not require that they follow the patient's wishes.

In a state where there is no such legislation, like Massachusetts, it would still be worthwhile for individuals to write down how they would wish to be treated if the time comes when they are incompetent to make such decisions, and to name someone who, in effect, would be the executor of the living will. By doing so, if decisions regarding that patient's care do get to court, the judge would have a very powerful indication of how that person would like to be treated under the circumstances.

Dr. Levine: My only, minor, disagreement with that is that we've asked people not to use the word "executor" in their living wills because of the serious peril of mispronouncing it.

Dr. James H. Gordon (Psychiatrist, Nassau County Medical Center, Great Neck, N.Y.): Concerning the issue of competence, who decides that? What about people who are not psychotic but deny that they have a problem or don't believe that such and such is going to happen? Practically, how do medical people handle that, and legally, how is the issue of competence determined?

Prof. Glantz: Competence is usually determined by a court. People are deemed to be competent unless they are proved to be incompetent. When people are found to be incompetent, they lose

the right to make certain decisions about themselves. I think that's
what Judge Liacos was talking about—that it is the role of the courts
to decide when someone loses the ability to make those decisions.
The courts don't make those determinations on their own; they rely
to a great extent on the medical profession. It usually requires a
finding of mental illness or great debilitation, something that
prevents a person from being able to understand what the situation
is and what the risks and benefits are. It's not enough that someone
else disagrees with the person or believes the person is making a
bad decision. There has to be some condition that prevents that
person from making judgments based on full information.

Prof. Murphy: I have a question about Dr. Levine's criteria. Are the
people who fall into your category of comfort measures removed or
banned from intensive care units? Many nurses are troubled when
they have orders not to use extraordinary measures or, more
commonly, not to resuscitate patients who are in intensive care
units. They feel that the purpose of the unit is to prolong life, to give
lifesaving treatment; if a patient is not there for that reason, there is
a conflict in philosophy.

Dr. Levine: That's a very serious problem. We were tempted to try
to resolve it through a policy recommendation, but we decided not
to. We finally suggested that receiving comfort measures only is not
an automatic reason for transfering a patient out of the intensive
care unit. A lot has to do with the facts of the particular situation.
Sometimes these people have developed their main support
community with personnel in the intensive care unit, and we
certainly would not want to break that off. On the other hand, if a
patient has been insentient during the entire stay in the unit, there's
not much support to break off. The toughest cases arise when we
have a full intensive care unit, including somebody who is not to be
resuscitated or to get other special devices, and somebody else
comes along who really needs all the expertise of the unit. That's
where we have our most anguishing decisions.

Prof. Murphy: If your program is implemented, what will happen
in terms of third-party payments—for example, when there is an
audit of a patient identified as being there for comfort measures
only, at the cost of hundreds of dollars a day for the bed?

Dr. Levine: That's one of the reasons I don't like to talk about nontreatment decisions. A decision to comfort patients is not a decision to discontinue treatment; rather, it is a decision to continue treatment of a different sort. Actually, there is a potential problem with some third-party payers. But it is very important that we recognize that we are not talking about abandoning a patient in any sense of the word. It is quite legitimate to call our comforting procedures medical treatment, and they are certainly worthy of third-party payment, although my opinions don't necessary prevail in the policy-making arena.

Mr. Freishtat: Let me return to some of the implications of the *Dinnerstein* case. *Dinnerstein* was the first appellate case in the nation to deal with do not resuscitate orders. Although Judge Liacos questioned whether the case even needed to be brought to court, I think many of us here are probably very glad that it was because it helped clarify some things. What it basically says is that do not resuscitate orders for terminally, irreversibly ill patients—the so-called hopeless cases—don't require prior judicial approval.

Let me move from a do not resuscitate situation to a situation of, say, withdrawal from a respirator. Assume that a competent patient or a once-competent patient made clear that only comfort measures should be administered; these measures have the incidental effect in some cases of shortening life, although that may not have been their intent. Assume that this person is now hopeless. Are the medical or legal considerations different from the do not resucitate situation? Based on the present state of medicine and law, do these cases need to be brought to court for prior judicial approval?

Dr. Prout: We've made it easy for ourselves by talking about the extremes. We've talked about resuscitation as a full-blown cardiopulmonary resuscitation. More commonly, the type of situation I see is where I want a patient in a unit for monitoring of arrhythmias, because I will treat arrhythmia, but I do not want to intubate the patient, because that will stimulate bleeding as a result of the cancer in the lung, and it is the cancer that I'm treating. There are all kinds of gradations. Legal precedents are set at the extremes, and we live in the middle. We have to make individual judgments about many such senarios, from monitoring and treating arrhythmias, to giving or not giving an intravenous, to encouraging someone to eat who wants to starve to death. I don't expect a lot of legal help for our decisions, except from the extremes.

Prof. Glantz: From the facts that you gave, Mr. Freishtat, I would ask why the patient is on the respirator. I believe you are referring to a person who is now incompetent, but was once competent, and when competent, requested not to be put on a respirator. Now someone wants to withdraw the respirator. I don't see the distinction between withdrawing and withholding, although many people do. If the withdrawing occurs in exactly the same circumstances under which you would have withheld treatment, had that been within your power, I don't believe the law would make a distinction.

Actually, the law has left this area alone; there is no case dealing with the withdrawal of treatment in that way. As far as we know, no physician has been sued and no criminal prosecution has been brought. This area has been left alone, and probably rightfully so, for the moment.

Mr. Russ Brown (Graduate student, Hospital Administration Program, Yale University, New Haven, Conn.): My question concerns dialysis patients. I have recently completed a 12-year retrospective study for the End-Stage Renal Disease Federal Coordinating Council in Connecticut. We found that approximately 2 percent of the 1,500 patients chose to discontinue dialysis and died. How do you counsel family members who have philosophical, theological, and financial concerns about such a decision? Sometimes, family members did not want dialysis discontinued because of the uncertainty as to whether it would be considered an act of suicide. For some families, the difference may mean a lot theologically. For others, it matters financially, because of life insurance.

Dr. Prout: When somebody has a chronic, incurable disease and has decided that therapy is worse than the alternative, which is death, it is the patient's right to discontinue the therapy. Now, for the legal aspect, as I read the law, that's not suicide. This comes up often when patients want to stop chemotherapy, and dialysis is no picnic, despite those who say that it's easier than chemotherapy. I believe that patients who have elected to discontinue treatment have made a very informed choice and a real value judgment.

When the family resists this choice, I try to get the family members to come in during the treatment so that they can see the toxicities. This has been pretty successful in giving them a greater appreciation for the suffering that's involved. We can also give the family pastoral counseling, psychiatric or psychiatric nursing counseling, and other kinds of support. Mostly, though, it's important that they see the treatment and have some kind of estimate of the toxicity.

Dr. Levine: Patients sometimes think that there is a moral constraint imposed on them by their religion, which may only reflect a misunderstanding of what their religion calls for. Depending on what the religion is, it might be quite proper to bring in a member of the clergy to explain what the real expectations are. Under the circumstances described, I am not aware of any theologians or clergy who would consider a decision to discontinue dialysis to be the moral equivalent of suicide. If I understood what Prof. Glantz said earlier, it doesn't seem to be the legal equivalent of suicide, either. I believe that this is one area where you can advise family members that at least one of the problems they are concerned with can be bypassed. Now, the second problem is whether the insurance company will consider it suicide. If legally it's not suicide but the insurance company decides that it is, I suppose you'd have to go to court.

Mr. Freishtat: Recognizing the tendency of insurance companies to read their contracts fairly tightly, I would guess that it might make a difference whether the withdrawal from dialysis took place at home, on the one hand, in a hospital, on the other, or maybe in a hospice, in between. To the extent that it occurred in a hospital, there might be more grounds for claiming that it was not an act of suicide and more of a way to document that fact than if it took place at home. That may be contrary to a lot of other moral and just considerations of appropriateness, but that is my initial reaction.

Prof. Glantz: Many living will laws contain a clause that if a person dies as a result of the enforcement of a living will, it is not to be deemed suicide for insurance reasons. Also, there is one case in which a Jehovah's Witness, who became disabled after refusing to consent to a transfusion, was found not to have self-inflicted the harm; whether the person was able to collect disability insurance as a result is still unsettled.

THE INCOMPETENT PATIENT: RIGHTS AND RESPONSIBILITIES

II

Problems of Uncertainty: Medical Criteria in Neonatal Treatment Decisions

I. David Todres, M.D.

Medical decisions about treatment are often concerned with the future quality of life. In a newborn, this is a special concern, because we are talking about an infant who is going to develop into an adult and possibly live for 70 years or more. When physicians look at statistics relating to treatment, they need to consider not only mortality but also morbidity—that is, the quality of survival. In the newborn, when we debate this quality of survival, it is usually because of the likelihood of a mental or physical handicap or both. At the outset, we must recognize that quality of life is a value judgment that is relative to the person making that judgment.

　　Let me cite two examples to demonstrate relative value judgments as they occur in the newborn. In our newborn intensive care unit, we cared for a very premature baby who was barely hanging onto life and required the use of a respirator to help the infant sustain breathing. The baby developed the severe complication of a hemorrhage into the brain. The parents expressed great concern about the severe and damaging brain hemorrhage. Both parents were university professors and looked at the situation from the point of view of the child's future intellectual development. They were very concerned that if this child survived and was severely mentally handicapped, life for the child might not be worth living. That is one perspective.

My second example is a baby born with abnormalities, which included the absence of an arm. The baby, otherwise, appeared well. A few days after birth, the infant developed breathing difficulties that required the use of a respirator. Although the family was obviously worried about the child's well-being and anxious about the outcome, the parents focused mostly on the infant's lack of an arm. In talking with us, they expressed the concern that the child would not be able to function well physically because of its handicap. The father was a farmer; he saw a stigma in a child who would not be able to work physically on the land, as previous generations of his family had all been able to do. There was no focus on the potential intellectual ability of the child.

These two examples illustrate the complexity of quality-of-life judgments in considering the care of the sick newborn.

In the last decade, we have brought a great deal of technology to the care of the newborn. We can now save many infants who otherwise would have died. But technology has also introduced new dilemmas, which continue to plague us. We have the knowledge and skill to use these new devices, but we may well ask whether we have the wisdom to use them.

As an example of the problems of uncertainty we face in caring for the newborn, let me talk about infants with a condition called spina bifida, also known as meningomyelocele. In this condition, there is an absence of bony parts of the spine, with the result that part of the spinal cord and nerve elements protrude and lie outside the spinal canal. This results in the child's being paralyzed from the point of the lesion downward, often from the lower or middle back; such children are usually incontinent as well. A significant number of these infants also develop hydrocephalus, which in some cases may result in a mental handicap.

Spina bifida can be treated by means of an operation on the back. But many of the infants who survive do so with very severe handicaps, physical and sometimes also mental. In addition, the future life of the child is interrupted by numerous infections and surgical procedures. Some are rehabilitated to function well; others are confined to a wheelchair for life.

Several years ago, Dr. John Lorber from England, working

with a team caring for these infants, established criteria to help physicians, nurses, parents, and others decide whether such a child should or should not be treated. He chose five criteria, one of which was that an infant with a particular degree of abnormality would not survive and should therefore not be treated. At that time, making a decision not to treat certain infants was a totally new approach; previously, surgeons had routinely operated on and treated these children, hoping for the best possible outcome. Dr. Lorber took a bold step when he set up these criteria — introducing an approach that was bound to provoke intense discussion and marked differences of opinion. Gerald Leach, in his book *Biocrats*, said, "Active treatment is the easy way out; most of us don't have the moral courage to think of other approaches."

Dr. Lorber's team and other groups followed this selective treatment approach for a number of years. What they discovered was that not all those infants who fitted into the nontreatment category died shortly after birth, as was anticipated. A number went on to survive several years. Some of these babies remained severely paralyzed, developed severe hydrocephalus, and were blind and deaf. The complications became extremely difficult to manage. Questions concerning what could have been done that could have altered their course then arose. Would an operation at the beginning of or during the child's early life have changed the sequence of events? This raised a lot of concern about the validity of drawing up criteria for a decision to treat or to withhold treatment.

Let me give another example. A 3-month-old infant with meningomyelocele was admitted to our hospital for further management. The baby had not received operative therapy at birth. Usually a decision to treat (i.e., to operate) is made within the first 24 hours. In this case, the parents had taken the child to a neurologist, whose impression was that the baby was severely handicapped and most unlikely to have any meaningful life whatsoever; the parents participated in a choice not to treat the infant. In the next three months, the child developed some ability to move, though very limited; the child also developed a personality, and an interaction between the parents and child was established. At this point, a second medical opinion was sought. The parents were now informed that examination of the infant showed a good chance that the child would do quite well. This opinion was confirmed by a neurologist, who suggested operative therapy, and an operation was performed at the request of the parents. The dilemma here is that this child subsequently has not done so well as had been hoped, and the question is whether the child would have done better had treatment started right from the beginning.

In treatment decisions, we are faced with a dilemma because results of therapy or nontherapy are often uncertain. In setting up criteria, we try to establish what the probabilities are. We are always going to have a certain degree of error in our judgment. And in the very young, the degree of certainty is very fallible. The newborn has not lived a life from which we can make presumptions about the future. Charles Nicolle, the distinguished French bacteriologist, addressed the fallibility of physicians and our decisions many years ago when he said, "All method is imperfect. Error is all around it, and at the least opportunity, it invades it. But what can we do? There is no other way."

Another difficulty in medicine concerns the interpretation of statistical data. When we talk in terms of data and survival statistics, we are still uncertain as to the outcome for the individual child we are treating. As far as the parents, physicians, and nurses are concerned, statistics make it difficult to use treatment or nontreatment criteria in a particular case.

One reason that the criteria are so very difficult to interpret is that the criteria themselves have been developed according to the results of treatment carried out many years ago. We have to be very careful how we interpret them. As we look at the data regarding intensive care and newborns, for example, we need to recognize that the data reflect what existed 10 years ago or more. In the interim, the treatment is likely to have changed so much that what actually happened 10 years ago is not relevant to present management decisions.

The improving prognosis is in large measure due to sophisticated medical technology. While technology has provided many solutions to the problems of the sick newborn, it has also been responsible for creating new problems. It is important, however, to see technology as a means of helping us resolve some of these dilemmas of life. Let us look at a specific example, namely, the use of the recently developed computed tomography scanner technique, also known at the CT scan.

The majority of babies in the intensive care unit are very premature neonates or infants with very low birth weights. A great many of these babies also have respiratory difficulties, and in the past, many of them died as a result. Now we are able to care for them, and death from respiratory difficulties is far less common than it was in the past. However, what often happens to these infants, unfortunately, is that they sustain a brain hemorrhage, which often leads to their deaths. Others survive but with permanent mental and physical handicaps. We then wonder whether we can set up criteria for nontreatment based on the degree of hemorrhage into the brain, considering the possibility that catastrophic brain hemorrhage with a hopeless outcome would not warrant ongoing intensive care. Thus, we are trying to use sophisticated technology to help us resolve some of the problems. For example, CT scan machines can now "look into" the brain and measure the extent of the hemorrhage. We are able to look at infants who sustain this tragic event and predict, not with certainty but with reasonable accuracy, how this child may develop in the future according to the extent of the hemorrhage. Through technology, now we are able to do something previously not possible. Technology thus may balance new problems with new solutions.

I would like to close with some words of wisdom that came from a physician and a philosopher 800 years ago; it is most applicable to what we are discussing today. Maimonides said:

> Just as there is a limit to the use of man's physical powers, there is a limit to the use of the intellectual powers. Too much speculation and scientific investigation can exhaust a man's intellect and lead to doubt and confusion. Sometimes it is good to admit doubt and acknowledge that not everything can be absolutely proved. If you come to this point of development, you have reached the pinnacle of human perfection. But if you reach beyond human comprehension or deny methods that have never been truly disproved or which are in fact remotely possible, then you might end up confused, imperfect, skeptical, and flawed.

Treatment Decisions and Triage: The Physician's Burden

Benson B. Roe, M.D.

7

The remarkable achievements of medical technology in the past two to three decades have created serious socioeconomic problems that weigh heavily against their benefits in terms of preservation or improvement of human life. Life expectancy at birth has, indeed, been significantly extended by nearly obliterating infant and childhood mortality from infectious disease. The life expectancy of the American male in late middle age, however, has been extended by only eight-tenths of a year in the last century—despite an enormous outpouring of medical technology at an incalculable cost in dollars, effort, and suffering.

It is distressing that our efforts in the educational process and in the clinical literature to emphasize the humanitarian aspects of health care have done so little to budge modern physicians from their crusade to slay the dragon of death. In the days when the grim reaper was omnipotent, physicians recognized the futility of defiance and gracefully confined their services to providing comfort, solace, and support. Today, we have at hand—and therefore feel obliged to use—an impressive armamentarium of exceedingly expensive life-support systems that are capable of fending off the natural process of dying for days, weeks, or even months. For example, antibiotics prolong terminal pneumonias; respirators sustain breathing beyond the patient's capacity to sustain life independently; dialysis averts the fatal consequences of destroyed kidneys; and balloon systems and pumps keep the blood circulating when the heart can no longer do it.

These huge undertakings create heavy burdens with which we must reckon. The financial burden must be borne either by a desperate and perhaps bankrupt family or by premium-paying insurance subscribers and taxpayers. How many of us will derive even a few happy additional hours in return for our share of this growing burden? The emotional burden of this elaborate treatment is often devastating to both patient and relatives; and regrettably, it tends to be compounded by an unjustified hope. Are the results commensurate with the emotional price? The physical burden (of misery) must be borne by the helpless patient, who may wish none of the suffering or even the life that is being preserved.

It is gross negligence for physicians to ignore, or even to minimize, these burdens, but they rationalize them as part of the necessary, and therefore acceptable, price for "saving a life." What is more, our societal attitudes have made it an atrocity to let anyone die for lack of money or effort even in the face of a very limited life expectancy. The physician's creed has, therefore, become "Damn the expense—full speed ahead!"

Up to now, this has been the prevailing attitude. Our national wealth is enormous; our compassion is boundless; and the anemic taxpayer has not yet turned into a turnip. But it simply cannot continue much longer. We have all seen the precipitous ascent of health costs that have quadrupled, in real dollars, in less than 30 years and now consume 9 percent of the Gross National Product. The geometric growth of scientific technology promises to continue, and the capability to maintain some semblance of life almost indefinitely is certainly not far off. Artificial hearts will soon be available, at $30,000 per item; kidney dialyzers, respirators, oxygenators, and a host of other machines are already used to replace the functions of other vital organ systems.

The technical possibilities are infinite; if we can send people to the moon, we certainly can conquer the biological problem of artificially sustaining life. The difficulty, however, is that we do not have the economic and sociological capability to support such a project beyond the laboratory stage, just as it is not feasible to hold conventions on the moon. Our health care resources, though vast, are not unlimited, and their expenditure will have to be restrained. There are not enough physicians or enough dollars to provide every dying patient with indefinite total technological support.

Thus, we turn to the subject of treatment decisions and how they are to be made. The outcomes of these decisions affect the patients, their families, and the rest of society, all of whom have some right and responsibility to participate. When patients are alert, stable, and intelligent, it is sufficient and appropriate that they and their personal physicians consider the alternatives and make the choices together. When patients are not capable of this responsibility, it may be appropriate for their families to act as surrogates.

Nevertheless, circumstances do arise that frequently prevent some patients from making an objective decision. For example, the perspective of a suffering patient may be distorted by pain, despair, fear, and scientific ignorance; the disease may cloud judgment. The symptoms and emotional distress may be unbearable enough for a patient to insist on being allowed to die, even though the disease is curable. On the other hand, a patient may be misled by a blind faith in the power of the physicians or the treatment itself. Indeed, instinct for survival may drive someone beyond the vast resources of scientific medicine to seek out worthless potions from fraudulent quacks in the vain hope of a cure.

Family members have complex emotional ties that may make them even less qualified to carry the responsibility for treatment decisions. A feeling of guilt may generate a denial of the inevitability of death and provoke them to insist irrationally on doing everything possible to save "dear old Dad." Conversely, they may detest him for his demanding and parsimonious ways or be exasperated over the burden of his chronic care, and thus they may welcome the prospect of his demise. Furthermore, their grasp of the scientific background may be insufficient to provide a realistic understanding of the available options and their impact on treatment.

Management of the human life in jeopardy properly rests with trained professionals whose background, experience, and psyche have prepared them to make these difficult decisions and to deal with the consequences when they are occasionally wrong. They must not be intimidated by the critic who challenges a decision on the basis of some unlikely anecdote. It is the responsibility of physicians to determine how patients wish to live and what they wish to endure and to protect them against the hazards of incompetence, carelessness, and fraud.

Certainly, the desires of patients who wish to undertake a risk or are unwilling to exceed a minimal level of discomfort must be respected in the decision-making process. But physicians are responsible for interpreting these desires in realistic terms of treatment, for educating those involved, and for guiding the events that will lead to the ultimate satisfaction of both the patients and their families. Physicians cannot pass the buck to a committee, to a family, or even to a patient. In my opinion, this responsibility has been neglected; I believe that peer pressure, legal reprisal, and a sheer lack of guts have resulted in a cop-out in this area. California's recently enacted Natural Death Act is in part an expression of this failure and a condemnation of overextended medical practices.

Part of the problem lies in the unwillingness of many physicians to grapple with the psychological challenges of the dying patient and in the convenient alternative of substituting technology for compassion. Another part of the problem, particularly in major academic centers, lies in the professional competition for results and the concept that losing a patient may reflect failure. And perhaps, if I were to be cynical, part of the problem even lies in the economic gain from extended heroics.

The "devoted physician"—depicted fretting at a sick child's bedside in the American Medical Association's propaganda poster of the 1960s, technically helpless, comforting, and hopeful of God's grace—is now replaced by a space age scientist. No longer can physicians hide behind the medical outcome as being "God's will." Physicians are deeply involved in the course of events, and they carry the responsibility for applying and distributing the resources of their profession. It is time for them to recognize that these resources are not unlimited, that humans are not immortal, and that peace and comfort should be their primary objectives. They must accept without guilt the validity of decisions to withhold or withdraw treatment. Physicians should be charged with improving the quality of life, instead of its simple quantity. Death in orgiastic ecstasy is worth a decade of dotage terminated in pitiful, impotent misery.

The concept of selective treatment, after all, is not new. Wartime triage, born of necessity, worked very well in the best interests of the whole. Wounded soldiers were distributed into three pathways. First, the hopelessly destroyed, whose chances of survival were remote and whose individual treatment would consume the time and resources to treat a score of others, were set aside to die as comfortably as possible with medication. Second, the salvageable patients in critical need of medical care to survive and recover were given the full measure of medical capability, with a fantastic record of success in our three most recent wars. The third category included the salvageable patients who could safely wait for medical attention until they were returned to the station hospital and still survive without serious consequence.

This process of distributing patients for treatment recognized the reality of limited capabilities and resulted in an optimal concentration of effort and resources on those who would ultimately benefit the most, with minimal disservice to others. It worked. And the time has come for us to incorporate these principles into civilian medicine. The heavy responsibility of deciding which patients to remove from the treatment pathway has enormous ramifications— moral, legal, and scientific—that we must promptly address.

The role of playing God may be uncomfortable, but it is not without precedent in our society. We accept decisions made by judges, generals, airline pilots, engineers, and public health officials, some of which also involve life and death. The logistics of dealing with this problem are not simple. Sometimes the choices are easy, and the outcome is certain one way or another. Sometimes expectations are favorable at the outset, only to deteriorate into hopelessness. And at other times, it can be almost frightening to encounter unexpected recovery from what had seemed to be an unsalvageable state.

Unfortunately, however, we have not learned to cope with patients whose hopeless states can be recognized only after they are already involved in an advanced stage of therapeutic commitment, such as accident victims who are resuscitated from a moribund state and sustained in intensive care, or postoperative patients whose operations were more devastating than expected and for whom recovery is unlikely. To withdraw support deliberately under these circumstances is far more difficult than it would have been to withhold the treatment initially. It is this group of patients, however, on whom our attention must be focused in the current discussion and for whom physicians need help.

It is obvious that physicians cannot assume the full responsiblity for these patients, in the sense that I have advocated, because of legal and social restraints. Nevertheless, I charge physicians with moral and professional obligations to provide a knowledgeable, balanced, mature recommendation and to present it with reason, conviction, and determination, so that it will prevail over irrational controversy or emotional challenge. To assist physicians in carrying this burden for our mutual benefit, I challenge the legislature, the judiciary, the clergy, and the sociologists with providing supportive mechanisms.

Treatment and Nontreatment Decisions: In Whose Best Interests?

Judith P. Swazey, Ph.D.

8

My concern with the nature of treatment and nontreatment decisions has been from the perspective of someone who wandered into bioethics from biology and the history and sociology of medicine. As such, I have worked chiefly as a descriptive ethicist, interested in analyzing the discourses of normative ethicists, medical professionals, lawyers, and policymakers.

A major theme in the rapidly growing literature on treatment and nontreatment determinations and in the actual decision-making process is how the related concepts of best interests and value or quality of life ought to enter into such decisions. Whether and on what bases competent adults should make their own treatment decisions is one segment of the debate. This debate grows even more complex and unsettled as it turns to those who, medically or legally, cannot speak for themselves—incompetent adults and minors.

If we agree, ethically, with the view of the Massachusetts Supreme Judicial Court in the *Saikewicz* decision that the right of competent patients to refuse treatment must be extended to incompetent persons as well, because "the value of human dignity extends to both," we then must deal with such questions as who ought to exercise the incompetent patient's right to refuse treatment and what criteria ought to be used. Traditionally, nontreatment decisions for incompetent patients have been exercised by physicians and family or guardians, with varying degrees of collegiality in the decision-making process. The focus of decision making, however, increasingly is shifting to the courts, frequently moved there, at least initially, by the traditional decision makers themselves.

Before exploring the "who and how" of these decisions, I would argue that, whoever the decision makers are, they should define their moral role as that of a steward, one who manages another's affairs and, in so doing, presumably acts in that person's best interests. Ethically, the least ambiguous role for stewards is in handling the affairs of incompetent patients who had once been competent and had used an instrument such as a living will to express their treatment preferences should they become voiceless. In such cases, it seems to me, the steward's moral obligation is to act nonpaternalistically according to what once-competent patients had defined as their own best interests, whether or not it is a course of action with which the steward agrees.

If the incompetent patient is a newborn or never-competent adult, the steward's role, both morally and practically, is less well charted, for there is no patient-drawn map of best interests to follow. In this situation, stewards can elect to do what they think is in the patient's best interests, based on judgments as to what most competent people would choose to do or what they themselves would choose. This is at once the most strongly paternalistic and the most ambiguous and elastic sort of determination of best interests, one that, properly or not, can let a variety of interests enter into the decision-making matrix.

A more weakly paternalistic stewardship role is the exercise of what is legally called substituted judgment, as adopted by the Massachusetts Supreme Judicial Court on behalf of Joseph Saikewicz. In exercising substituted judgment, stewards, by admittedly complex feats of mental gymnastics, try to reason what incompetent patients would deem to be in their own best interests if they were able to become briefly competent and assess their incompetent selves. The application of substituted judgment is a complex and controversial procedure, and many people feel it is only a "legal fiction" when used for never-competent persons, because it is impossible to ascertain what such persons think is in their own best interests.

A fuller understanding and exercise of the stewardship role, I believe, would help resolve the present moral, medical, and legal morass that engulfs nontreatment criteria, although it would not neatly and simply answer the whole set of problems.

The lack of clarity that surrounds even the most thoughtful efforts to formulate nontreatment criteria is illustrated by the attempts of a 1974 conference to develop a moral policy for newborn intensive care. The conferees, for example, unanimously agreed that there are circumstances under which it would be "right to withdraw life support from a clearly diagnosed, poor prognosis infant." In then attempting to specify the "limiting conditions" for such decisions, the participants listed criteria within three categories: the child's situation (general physical status, general "human" status, and medical indications), the family situation, and miscellaneous factors.

However, the participants failed to explicate the value assumptions underlying their proposed criteria and to distinguish the various sets of interests that the criteria represent. This failure is exemplified by the criteria listed under general human status. The first criterion, most would agree, is directed toward the infant's best interests; life support may be withdrawn if the infant "will most probably be without self-awareness or socializing capacities." But the fourth criterion deals with judgments about the value of life and social worth that reflect interests far beyond the infant's; life support may be withdrawn "if the infant is defective and unwanted by its parents and unneeded by society."[1]

As this example suggests, many best interests can indeed be entered into a decision-making matrix. But if principled decisions are to be made, either in individual cases or for categories of cases, the actors first need to reach some consensus as to whose interests ought to be considered, in what order, by what indices, and within what limits. Arguments abound for and against considering the best interests of parties other than the patient. These other interests include the parents' willingness to care for a "defective" infant or child at home, the possible adverse effects (psychological, social, or economic) on the family of treating (or not treating) an "anomalous newborn" or prolonging the life of a comatose parent, the economic costs to the family or society of institutional care for a "salvaged" patient, the priorities of caring for patients with more favorable prognoses in medical facilities with limited resources, the relieving of stresses on the part of the staff caring for "hopeless" cases, or the nature of the physicians' professional responsibilities.

The use of these sorts of criteria for determining best interests for nontreatment decisions is controversial, particularly as they explicitly or implicitly involve judgments about the social worth or value of a voiceless patient's life. However, if only because criteria such as costs to society or adverse effects on the family are manifestly in the best interests of others than the incompetent person, they are easier to deal with than are efforts to define what really is in the incompetent patient's best interests. If we agree that the patient's best interests should be the primary, if not exclusive, consideration in nontreatment decisions, how do we determine what those interests are, and how do we guard against the intrusion of other interests?

Most efforts to define the best interests of an incompetent patient are couched in phrases that relate to the quality of life that individual would have with or without a given medical intervention. These judgments may be assessed in terms of what others feel are tolerable or intolerable physical deficits or in terms of cognitive functioning; this latter assessment is usually thought to be more central in quality-of-life considerations. Criteria regarding the quality of life have been discussed most frequently with respect to newborn intensive care, and here the criteria most often evoked echo the "indicators of humanhood" formulated in 1972 by utilitarian ethicist Joseph Fletcher.[2] Pediatrician Raymond Duff, for example, has observed that "the notions of humanhood stated by Fletcher are widely applied by families and physicians," and he discusses how his unit employs quality-of-life criteria that range from neocortical function to an infant's capacity to love and be loved, to be independent, and to understand, anticipate, and plan for the future.[3]

Other commentators, such as theologian Paul Ramsey, object on a priori ethical principles to the use of what they deem to be such value-laden quality-of-life criteria. Ramsey instead advocates using a "medical indication" policy in treatment or nontreatment decisions; for example, if surgery to correct duodenal atresia is medically indicated, it should be performed whether or not the infant has Down's syndrome. One problem with Ramsey's position is the arguable assumption that medical indications are value free. A second problem is that Ramsey goes on to discuss treatment decisions in terms of a patient's "potentiality for significant personal life," for "interrelationship with other human beings," and for "some relationship with God,"[4] criteria that surely are hard to fit within a medical indication policy.

As the foregoing examples suggest, quality- or value-of-life terms and arguments in relation to best interests are generally vague and are used in many ways and contexts. For these reasons, coupled with the difficulties of ensuring that such criteria are being put forth in the incompetent patient's best interests, the courts have been reluctant to permit their use in nontreatment decisions except under stringently narrow definitions.

The Massachusetts probate court and Supreme Judicial Court struggled with these quality- and value-of-life issues and distinctions in the case of Joseph Saikewicz. One factor that the probate court weighed was the quality of life possible for him even if the treatment did bring about remission. The Supreme Judicial Court held that "to the extent that this formulation equates the value of life [of Mr. Saikewicz as a retarded person] with any measure of the quality of life, we firmly reject it."[5] However, the court said that if quality of life refers to the continuing state of pain and disorientation precipitated by the chemotherapy, then it could be considered. It is this latter interpretation that the court adopted, within the framework of a substituted-judgment test. In looking at why and how the court utilized this particular, narrow, quality-of-life criterion, it is important to remember that the issue it was addressing was not whether to allow an incompetent patient to die as a result of nontreatment. Rather, the court was dealing with the manner of Mr. Saikewicz's dying—that is, with the quality of life he would experience with and without treatment for a disease that would inexorably end his life.[6]

Among pre-*Saikewicz* cases that also have implicitly or explicitly dealt with the issue of quality or value of life is the 1974 case of *Maine Medical Center* v. *Houle*, involving a blind newborn who had no left ear, some nonfused vertebrae, and some brain damage.[7] She also had a tracheoesophogeal fistula that was curable and would have caused her death without its repair. Her parents argued against treatment because of the poor quality of life the child would have if cured of her life-threatening condition. The court, however, held that the only issue to be decided was the medical feasibility of the procedure. If the procedure could not save her life, it need not be done; but if an otherwise healthy child required such surgery and if it would normally be done for such a child, then the fact that a child was blind, deaf, or retarded could not be taken into account.

The *Quinlan* court, in turn, used a very narrow quality- or value-of-life criterion, maintaining that if there was no reasonable possibility of Karen Quinlan returning to a cognitive, sapient state, the respirator sustaining her life could be turned off.[8] This is a value judgment that says that a person who is not cognitive or sapient need not be treated. It is, moreover, a judgment that the court did not couch in terms of what might or might not be in her best interests.

Houle, Quinlan, and *Saikewicz* offer different approaches to the use of value-of-life and quality-of-life criteria in nontreatment decisions. *Houle* seems to claim that when something medical can be done, it should be done. The *Saikewicz* case specifically rejects the use of value-of-life or social-worth criteria, although it does allow the use of quality-of-life criteria that pertain to the pain and suffering therapeutic intervention might cause. The *Quinlan* case implicitly permits the use of a very narrow value-of-life criterion that, though applied by the medical profession, was formulated by the judiciary. Although these approaches appear to be contradictory, it must be kept in mind that the decisions were based on very different factual circumstances and that a court's primary purpose is to resolve the particular conflict before it.

The at-once medical, ethical, social, and legal issues that we are exploring address the broader question of whether we can find bases and modes for making principled treatment or nontreatment decisions that will fall between the extremes of moral absolutism and ad hoc situational responses. Nontreatment decisions, Sister Margaret Farley has written, "are a problem only for those who consider all human life to be valuable and who nonetheless consider human physical life to be relative to other values. These latter ask what is human life relative to? What are the values for the sake of which human physical life can be let go? What are the values which, if they are missing, cease to ground a moral claim to human life in this world?"[9]

How to determine these values and to find acceptable means of acting on them is increasingly a matter of high public visibility and concern, and the more such decision making comes "out of the closet," the more evident are the substantive and procedural issues that await clarification and resolution.

REFERENCES

1.   Jonsen, A. R., and Garland, M., eds. *Ethics of newborn intensive care.* San Francisco and Berkeley: University of California School of Medicine and Institute of Government Studies, 1976, pp. 185–187.

2.   Fletcher, J. F. Indicators of humanhood: a tentative profile of man. *Hastings Cent. Rep.* 2:1–4, 1972; Four indicators of human-hood—the inquiry matures, *ibid.,* 4:4–7, 1974.

3.   Kelsey, B. Shall these children live? A conversation with Dr. Raymond S. Duff. *Hastings Cent. Rep.* 5:5–8, 1975; Duff, R. S., and Campbell, A. C. M. Moral and ethical dilemmas in the special-care nursery. *N. Engl. J. Med.* 289:890–894, 1973.

4.   Ramsey, P. *Ethics at the edges of life.* New Haven: Yale University Press, 1978, p. 161.

5.   *Superintendent of Belchertown State School* v. *Saikewicz,* 370 N.E.2d 417 at 432 (Mass. 1977).

6.   Glantz, L., and Swazey, J. Decisions not to treat: the *Saikewicz* case and its aftermath. *Forum on Medicine* 2:22–32, 1979.

7.   *Maine Medical Center* v. *Houle,* Maine Sup. Ct., Civ. Action No. 74–145 (1974).

8.   *In the Matter of Karen Quinlan,* 70 N.J. 10, 355 A.2d 647 (1976).

9.   Farley, M. Quoted in *Hastings Cent. Rep.* 5:6, 1975.

The Courts and Nontreatment Criteria

John A. Robertson, J.D.

9

The key to understanding court decisions allowing nontreatment for incompetent patients, and the factor that is most often confused, is the basic distinction between substantive and procedural criteria for nontreatment. The distinction was confused in the *Saikewicz* case and in the subsequent reaction to it, causing much of the resulting controversy about the decision.

Substantive criteria for nontreatment are criteria that define a class or group of patients from whom necessary medical care may be withheld. The class is specified in terms of mental functioning, physical conditions, or prognosis. In essence, the criteria represent a moral or social policy judgment that these states of being are not so important that we need expend further medical resources in providing them to the patient.

Procedural criteria, on the other hand, tell us how we must go about deciding whether a given patient falls within the group from whom medical care may be withheld. Procedural criteria concern the old questions of who shall decide and how it shall be decided, but they do not address the question of what shall be decided. One reason for setting procedural criteria is to make sure that the substantive criteria are applied correctly. They are a further protection for the patient and society.

The choice of both substantive and procedural criteria involves policy judgments, but different policy considerations apply to each. The choice of substantive criteria to define the class of patients from whom necessary care may be withheld is logically separate and involves a totally different set of policy considerations from those required for choosing the procedure to determine whether a patient falls within that category.

Concerning substantive criteria for nontreatment, we are currently in the midst of a minor legal revolution. Within the last few years, in such notable cases as *Quinlan, Saikewicz,* and *Dinner-stein,* the courts have begun to enunciate and articulate substantive grounds for withholding medical care that could extend life from persons who are incompetent and unable to express their views about it. In reading these opinions, it is interesting to note that they are directed to such questions as what is the best interest of this patient? What will benefit this patient? What would this patient want if he or she could somehow come out of incompetency and speak to us? The substantive criteria specified in these cases are patient-centered. They focus on the patient's needs and interests and not on the interests or concerns that doctors, family, and society have in whether or not treatment should occur.

The emphasis on patient-oriented substantive criteria is very reassuring. It enables everyone to function more easily, for it seems to say that if nontreatment—and, hence, an earlier death than is necessary—is to occur, it is to be done for the sake of the patient. It allows us to say that in withholding essential care from incompetent patients, we are respecting their rights; we are respecting their persons; and we are acknowledging the sanctity of their lives and their need to be treated fairly. We are not merely sacrificing patients who are powerless to protect themselves in order to benefit others.

I see significant problems, however, with the way in which the courts have applied the patient-centered substantive criteria that have been articulated. To develop and apply such criteria is not easy. How can we really tell what is in a patient's interests in such extreme circumstances? Do the substantive criteria developed truly serve the patient's best interests? When do the burdens, pain, and indignity required to keep someone alive outweigh the benefits to that person of the extra time of being alive? Is it of greater benefit to stay alive for a few weeks more or to die now? Suppose someone is comatose but not terminally ill and could exist in that state for a long period of time; is it in that person's interests to stay in that state of being?

To answer these questions, we need to be clear about when extending the life of a terminally ill or disabled incompetent person is indeed a benefit for that individual and when it is not. Questions like this have moral and religious overtones. Mental incompetency alone is not determinative of whether it is in a patient's interests to go on living. If we are going to rely on patient-oriented nontreatment criteria, as the courts in these cases have begun to do, we need to develop a social consensus about whether, in fact, it is in a patient's interests to die when such states exist or whether it is more in that person's interests to go on living. If we ask these questions from the perspective of the patient alone and put aside all other considerations, including the interests of other people, I think we might get a very different view of what is in the patient's interests than we get from the courts in cases where they purport to apply patient-oriented substantive criteria for nontreatment.

In the *Quinlan* case, for example, the court held that incompetent individuals have a right to personal privacy, which includes the right to reject care. The court concluded that if Karen Quinlan could somehow speak, she would ask to be taken off the respirator because it would not be in her interests to stay on it. In other words, the court was saying that removing her from the respirator, and supposedly causing her death, would actually benefit her. But think about it. Is nontreatment really in her interest? She is unconscious and feels no pain, as far as we can tell. She is certainly unaware of the considerable suffering her family and others have been experiencing, and thus she has no interest in relieving their burdens. In addition there is a small, finite chance that she could recover, so keeping her alive for that reason might be a benefit to her, for it at least leaves open the possibility of recovery. This is not to say that Karen Quinlan has a very great chance of recovery, but even a very small possibility suggests that it may be in her interests to continue to be alive. There is also another argument as to why Ms. Quinlan might wish to be kept alive, if she could tell us how to protect her interests. Some people believe that, because of their rapid eye movements, comatose individuals dream and therefore might be experiencing some state of being that is good in itself. Obviously, we do not know very much about this, but it is a consideration. In sum, a strict analysis of Ms. Quinlan's situation from her perspective alone leads to the conclusion that, far from being in her interests to be taken off the respirator, it is clearly in her interests to stay on it.

In the *Dinnerstein* case, the judge's opinion seems to rest on the notion that it is not in a terminally ill patient's interests to go on living or to be resuscitated again and again so as to gain additional days of life. Although there are circumstances in which that may be true, I do not believe that it is invariably so. In fact, the court implies that even a year of additional life for a terminally ill patient does not serve the interests of that person. Continued existence might not have served Mrs. Dinnerstein's interests, but it might well serve the interests of other terminally ill patients.

A difficulty arises, however, if we rigidly take the patient's interests as the standard for nontreatment. A strict interpretation of those interests will mean that we must continue to treat and keep the patient alive in many situations that entail large burdens on others. Continued treatment might prolong the suffering of the family; it might clash with the moral notions of doctors and nurses; and it might cost society a lot of money. Yet, from the patient's perspective, strictly speaking, continued life even in a diminished state, as an analysis of the *Quinlan* case shows, may well benefit that individual. We must ask, therefore, whether treatment required to serve the patient's interests can ever be withheld to serve nonpatient interests, and if so, under what circumstances.

This is the challenge that the courts and legislatures are going to have to face very soon. The hard part will be defining the circumstances in which the gain to the patient is so small that the heavy burden on others in providing it need not be undertaken. This will inevitably involve a utilitarian balancing, but I know of no other way to go about resolving the issue that gives due regard to everyone affected. Careful, constrained, and rigorous balancing of the conflicting interests is necessary to avoid the dangers inherent in some kinds of utilitarianism. The challenge will be for the courts and legislatures to maintain respect for the incompetent patient while responding to the social consensus that, on occasion, gives more weight to interests other than those of the patient.

Let me turn now to the procedural criteria. Suppose that the legislatures or the courts, in weighing the conflicting interests in nontreatment decisions, decide to promulgate substantive standards for withholding care. Suppose these standards give primary emphasis to the patient's interests, permitting care to be withheld only when it is clearly in the patient's interests, as I believe the *Saikewicz* and *Dinnerstein* courts tried to do. Or perhaps they go further and, in a narrow category of cases, permit nontreatment when the patient's interests are very small and the burdens of treatment on others are very great. (In my view, this is what happened in the *Quinlan* case, although it was not explicitly stated.) In such cases, legislators and judges must ask themselves the additional question of whether they should rely on the usual mode of privately initiated rule enforcement or whether they should define further procedures for applying the substantive criteria to individual cases.

Consider first the situation if no procedural criteria are added. If, as in *Quinlan* or *Saikewicz*, the standard is to treat the patient unless the patient's best interests require otherwise, doctors and families will have a rule to follow. They will know that if they do not follow that rule, they are subject to sanctioning by the courts. Simply enunciating the rule, however, might not be a very effective way of actually changing or influencing the behavior of those who have to apply the substantive standard to actual cases. They might not be very familiar with the rule or may have trouble knowing what it requires in a given case. This could lead to errors in determining whether a patient falls into the nontreatment category. If we rely on the private system of rule enforcement alone, erroneous decisions will not be very visible. The chance that an erroneous application of the substantive rules will come to the attention of the courts, and therefore sanctions can be imposed, may not be very great. Merely enunciating the rule may not affect the behavior of physicians and others to any great extent. The usual mode of rule enforcement that relies on an individual's bringing a complaint will not work well here, and some patients will wrongly be deprived of care that they have a right to have.

If we want to reduce errors in application and bring about the actual behavior intended by the rules, it might be worthwhile to require that a certain procedure be followed whenever the rule is applied to a given case. This course would be justified, in my view, when the costs of the additional procedure are very small relative to the gain in the reduction of error that the additional procedure would provide. Indeed, I think that both the New Jersey Supreme Court in *Quinlan* and the Massachusetts Supreme Judicial Court in *Saikewicz* intuitively felt something of this sort. In both cases, they went one step further than merely defining substantive standards for withholding care. They both said that a certain procedure must be followed in applying those standards.

In the *Quinlan* case, the substantive standard was that if the patient has no reasonable possibility of recovering a cognitive or sapient state, the physician has no legal duty to provide medical care. The doctor could acquire immunity in making this decision if the prognosis is first confirmed by a hospital ethics committee. In other words, care can be withheld provided that a certain procedure is followed, a procedure established to minimize error and bias in applying the rule, so as to make sure that the patient actually fits into that class. The court could have imposed different procedural requirements, such as a judicial hearing or the signature of another doctor. However, the court wisely required confirmation by a hospital prognosis committee because the question was a medical judgment regarding the patient's prognosis.

The same distinction between substance and procedure explains *Saikewicz*. Here, the substantive standard was that nontreatment was suitable only if the patient, under the substituted-judgment rule, would choose nontreatment if the patient were able to speak. But rather than rely only on doctors and families to decide in a particular case what the patient would choose if the patient were able to speak, the court went further and required a procedure for applying that standard in given cases. In my opinion, that was a wise choice. Despite the relatively expensive and perhaps stressful nature of a court hearing, only that kind of dispassionate proceeding can ensure proper application of the substantive criteria of substituted judgment. No one at the physician or hospital level is as well equipped as the courts are to apply substituted judgment to patients in these circumstances.

I think that the consternation arising from *Saikewicz* is not that the court specified a judicial procedure for similar decisions, but rather that it included broad language suggesting that all treatment decisions involving incompetence should come to court. In my view, Massachusetts physicians would be justified in being disturbed by this ruling if that was, in fact, what the court meant. While some language in the opinion implies just that, a careful reading would show that it could not have been intended. In short, I do not believe that requiring all nontreatment decisions to come to the courts is a good approach, although for particular categories, it is highly desirable.

The need for additional procedural criteria will depend on the context and the kind of decision involved. Some decisions will require merely the application of relatively clear standards, for example, a standard that is translatable in medical terms; this occurred in the *Quinlan* case with the phrase "recovery of cognitive ability." If an additional process is essential in such cases to ensure the effectiveness of that standard, it may be a medically oriented process and may even take place after the fact and not before. In other cases, however, the standard may be more complex, and a nonmedical procedure for applying the criteria may be justified, as in *Saikewicz*. But it does not follow that if a nonmedical procedure is justified for some cases, the same procedure must be used in all cases.

In conclusion, lawmakers who devise the substantive norms for ordering the competing values in a nontreatment decision should also consider the second-level policy issue of whether to include a particular procedure as an adjunct to the substantive norms to ensure their implementation. If this distinction between substance and procedure can be kept clearly in view, judges and legislators can develop workable rules that optimally reconcile the interests of patients, families, physicians, nurses, and society in making decisions to withhold care from incompetent patients.

Discussion

Judith P. Swazey, Ph.D.,
Moderator

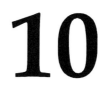

Prof. Swazey: I'd like to ask Dr. Todres and Dr. Roe to comment further on diagnostic uncertainty and treatment decisions. The problems of predictive uncertainty are clearly increasing, compounded by greater technological capabilities to keep people alive for longer and longer periods. Let's assume that we had a far more exact predictive capacity so that we could, for example, say with a fairly precise degree of certainty that the extent of the intraventricular bleed as measured by the CT scan means that this infant will have this degree of physical or mental impairment. Assume that we have the criteria and that the problems of uncertainty are no longer with us. Whom do you see as the people who most properly should look at the range of predictive criteria and say that these are the limits that we should adopt for a given decision either to intervene in some way or not to treat the infant at all? It's the same old question of who the decision maker should be, but with the predictive uncertainties hypothetically removed.

Dr. Todres: First, I must say that I don't think we are ever going to reach the point where we can be so certain of the criteria and have such accurate predictions that we will have clear-cut answers. A more common situation is one in which the physician says to the parents, "Your child has had a brain hemorrhage and will most likely be mentally and possibly physically abnormal, within a particular range. The child may be able to dress and feed itself, but I'm not quite sure about that." I run into this situation a lot. I think our predictive criteria are better than they were before. Our ranges were much broader in the past; we could give very little prognostic indication that could be narrowed down to certain situations and certain possibilities. We may be able to narrow it down even more, but I don't think we'll ever get to the point where we can be so precise as to say exactly what's going to happen. That's always going to be one of our dilemmas. I would hope that we can narrow it down to individual situations.

Regarding the question of decision making, I believe that the physician, who has the data and the experience as well as information on the progress of the particular infant, should present the data to the family, which is in the best position to speak for the infant. They can all sit down and discuss the situation and decide what to do. I think we have to make decisions in the context of the possible outcome of the particular patient. To be more specific than that, I'm afraid, will lead to a lot more trouble in the future.

Prof. Swazey: Do you think that decisions will essentially remain situational? In other words, for this infant and this set of parents, we need to consider these factors. Or do you think it is possible to make more broadly principled types of decisions?

Dr. Todres: Basically, when we talk about newborn infants, we're talking about three options. The first is to treat the infant with all possible resources: we can provide treatment; we have the machinery; we have the equipment for surgery; and there is no limit to what we do. The second option is to decide that the infant is so severely compromised that we won't treat this child; in fact, we might accelerate the child's death. The third option is to treat the child with the means at our disposal as long as we're helping the child in some way; but the time will come when we need to consider the quality of the infant's life, when we may not really be helping but rather hurting the child. Then the question comes up— how do we know when we're no longer helping the child? In other words, what's the outcome going to be? And here is where we get into the criteria of predictability. All we can do in this situation is share our information with the family and come to some mutual decision as to what we hope is in the best interest of that child. We include not only physicians and nurses but also the whole group of people who are taking care of the infant. We really can't do much better than that.

Dr. Roe: I'm concerned that we are so lacking in the courage to be wrong. We are dealing in an area of huge uncertainty, and we always have been. Just because we have a lot of information now that has reduced uncertainty in some areas does not mean that we can pretend that we are always going to be correct in what we recommend. But who is in a better position to make that overall assessment and recommendation than physicians? Let's recognize that we are not always going to be right for every individual, but this world already has a lot of people in it, and it's not as though life is that sacred. This country is unique, and this particular society is unique in its devotion to the sanctity of human life to the very remote fringes of its existence.

Dr. Prout: The patients that I talk with have greatly varying values of life and what constitutes for them adequate survival; many of them would want to have life-prolonging treatment. I've had patients tell me that they don't care if they end up just being able to go from the bed to a chair, or that they will be content just to watch the world go by, watch their grandchildren, or watch flowers — vegetate, as it were, or perhaps contemplate. These people can express these wishes because they are still cognitive. I find it very difficult to conceive of any way of applying these criteria to incompetent patients. I believe it is very arbitrary. I'm quite concerned about the implication that we as physicians can decipher values or have some kind of insight into what constitutes the value of life. I challenge our applying that. Physicians tend to use a cognitive value, and some use a physically functioning value as well, but neither of these is intrinsically adhered to by the patients themselves.

Dr. Roe: That's certainly a valid challenge. I guess that my position is to go back to square one and repeat that we are going to be wrong. I contend that we can be just as wrong by thinking that we are doing what the patient wants as we might be by being arbitrary.

The judgment of whether we are right or wrong is a very difficult one to make because it has overtones that involve not only the patient, but society at large, the patient's family, the economy, and a number of other things that we have alluded to. Thus, I do not find myself terribly concerned about taking the responsibility for these decisions, because I recognize that the forces of fate and nature over the quality and quantity of our lives are still far more vast than those that our profession is able to control. Since I can't compete with those forces, I don't have a very guilty conscience about the small amount that I may influence them in one direction or the other, if I do it in good faith for the sake of what I believe are the best interests of the patient and all those involved. I'm not disagreeing with you; I'm merely attempting to justify accepting that responsibility and to suggest that perhaps it is a kind of a charade to say that patients should have self-determination when I'm not so sure they even know what they really want.

Prof. Robertson: We are talking about the rules of the game, and the game is to decide which patients should get more medical care and which should not. The game concerns the allocation of medical care under circumstances in which it could have a very real effect on the patient, that is, could keep the patient alive. The question, then, is who should set the rules and who should decide which category of patients get the care and which do not. It seems to me that Justice Liacos said it as well as it can be said—that it is a societal decision for the designated societal decision makers, legislatures and courts, to make in an open way. In other words, these are nonmedical value and social policy questions that have to be answered by our nonmedical social policy organs. Then, within the rules laid down, it is up to the various doctors and others to apply them in particular circumstances. The underlying rules, however, must be socially designated because so much is at stake.

Prof. Swazey: Are you implying that the courts should set very specific criteria, as opposed to a broad procedural framework within which other elements in society, whether it is individuals or families or groups, decide more specifically?

Prof. Robertson: As I attempted to say earlier, someone has to set substantive criteria, such as which group of patients should not get further care, whether it is to advance the patients' own interests or whether it is a case in which the interests of others can justifiably be advanced at the patients' expense. Then the second question concerns the procedures to be used in a given case to decide whether an individual falls within that group. We have to keep those two concepts separate.

Dr. Todres: I am not comfortable with armchair decisions made away from the scene and away from reality. When we make decisions such as to set up rules, we imply that everybody gets fair treatment. Very often in an intensive care unit, great anguish is shared by physicians, nurses, parents, and every other person taking care of a particular child; there is enormous concern about that child's potential outcome. It is very difficult to fall back on rules that say either that this child should not get treatment and be left possibly to die or that this child must get very aggressive treatment and perhaps end up severely compromised. Meanwhile, society, whose responsibility it is, having set the rules, does a pretty poor job of taking care of such children outside the intensive care unit. It is hard to treat a sick infant and know that if you keep the baby alive, this baby will be severely compromised and will have to be institutionalized. Most of us sitting in armchairs and making these decisions haven't really seen these institutions, where in many cases the conditions are very far from satisfactory. So, I am uncomfortable with setting up rules unless society takes on the full burden of the obligations inherent in those rules.

Prof. Robertson: As one who tends to sit in an armchair and thus not be so closely involved as others are, I still maintain that this is a basic value choice that has to be faced. For example, why is it worse for a child to die rather than to live in a perhaps horrible institution? Conversely, why is it clear that a child, from its own perspective, is better off dead than alive in those circumstances? Also, we need not even go to extreme cases; we can talk about a fairly typical case. In many hospitals throughout America, a child with Down's syndrome who needs some fairly routine medical procedure to stay alive will not be provided with it simply because of the Down's syndrome and the fact that the child will be mildly or perhaps severely retarded. That kind of decision—that refusal of necessary medical care to someone solely because of a mental disability—is being made all the time. This is a nonmedical value judgment, and it's being made by doctors and families. It is situations like this for which the basic rules of the game need to be enunciated more clearly, so that they can be more easily applied in practice. Not all cases will be as easy as a child with Down's syndrome, but we can begin with that as an example of why rules are necessary.

Dr. Roe: Am I incorrect that this issue was settled legally as far back as the Kennedy administration, and that it is now illegal to deprive medical care to children afflicted with Down's syndrome?

Prof. Robertson: I would agree that it is illegal, but as I said earlier, privately initiated rule enforcement often does not work because many people don't know about the law, don't believe that such nontreatment is illegal, might think it's a good thing, and so on. Such a nontreatment decision may never come to the attention of the court. In fact, Dr. Todres's own survey of pediatricians in Massachusetts showed that a majority of the doctors would not repair a duodenal atresia on a Down's syndrome child if faced with that decision. That is the kind of nonmedical value judgment that we have effectively delegated to doctors and families. What is happening now is a reevaluation of whether we should continue delegating the responsibility to physicians to do as they see fit or whether we need some rules or constraints on the exercise of their discretion if we are to honor some rather basic values, such as respect for life and equality of everyone, regardless of such judgments as social worth or IQ. Now, in saying this, I admit that there is a point at which I, too, recognize that the gain to the incompetent patient may be so small and the burden on others so great that we are morally and socially justified in not requiring further care. I think that the debate should be over where to draw that line.

Dr. Roe: That is precisely the issue I attempted to introduce. Our whole discussion today has been predicated on the assumption that we have an unlimited capacity to take care of every vestige of life that's possible. We have operated on the basis that we have never not treated somebody because there is not enough to go around. But I am convinced that our technology and our costs are expanding at a rate where this totality is no longer feasible and that this situation will have to be faced realistically by someone. And that someone is all of us, not just physicians; physicians will have to give the opinions, but all of us will have to draw the guidelines and implement them. Obviously, the guidelines are going to be arbitrary, and wherever they're drawn, individual interpretations will put a particular patient on one side of them or the other. But we have to be able to grapple with the issue, and we have to have the courage to be wrong.

Prof. Robertson: You expressed the underlying dilemma very well. We do live in a world of scarcity, and we can't ignore it. The problem is in knowing how to deal with the fact of scarcity and how to decide who gets what. The traditional mode of allowing doctors and families to work out such decisions is simply not a very good way of going about it, wherein the parties decide according to their own heterogeneous views, which vary with who they are, where they are, what training they have had, and even how they feel on a given day. There is too much at stake for the individual patient, who might lose life itself as a result of an erroneous decision made for society as a whole.

Dr. Levine: Perhaps it would be perfectly proper to make decisions regarding classes of treatment or classes of procedures that may or may not be done on classes of people. But, Dr. Roe, you seem to have perceived a social injustice. As you talk with an individual patient or family member, do you ever take into account that by prolonging the life of that particular person, the overall economic burden to the state or the country may be increased? Is this a decision that you would personalize in a particular case?

Dr. Roe: No, because until now, I have shared the luxury of an economy in which such a decision has not been necessary. Having participated in triage, I recognize that it is a heavy burden, but it is one that can be dealt with, and the time is going to come when we will have to deal with it in civilian medicine. It will not be easy, and we may make tragic mistakes, but we have an overall responsibility to be able to say that treatment of patient A inevitably will result in the inability to treat unknown patient X, because we do have limitations. I don't know the answers to making the guidelines, and I think they are going to be very difficult, but we cannot keep sweeping the issue under the rug.

Dr. Levine: While I basically agree with you, I think that triage differs in very relevant ways from what usually goes on in civilian hospitals, unless it is a small town and a disaster occurs. Until guidelines for selecting among types of patients are articulated by society, I believe that it is not appropriate to enter societal costs into the individual decision-making arena, to calculate what's available for any particular patient. To that extent, I'd have to agree with Dr. Robertson.

Dr. Roe: I'm saying the same thing; we cannot do it now. However, society, the judiciary, and the legislature must develop guidelines so that we can do these things in the future.

Dr. Levine: But you seemed to be saying that physicians would have to assume the burden of making decisions and of perhaps being wrong and that the social costs might be one of the factors entering into the individual physician's burden.

Dr. Roe: Not in the current setting.

Dr. Prout: I have to disagree. We are already in an era of limited resources, at least where I work, and I'm afraid that social value is being used as a criterion for application of those resources. This setting is unlike the military setting, where everybody is perceived to be socially equal and ranking is done solely on the physical damage and the individual's ability to survive. Let me cite what happened during the 1978 blizzard in the Boston area when I tried to get an ambulance for one of my inner-city patients. This man had an advanced but controlled malignancy and was doing fine at home until he developed pneumonia. Because of the blizzard, we couldn't get nursing services to him, so I tried to get an ambulance. I was told that the ambulance service was only taking heart attacks, thank you. But, I found, cancer patients from the more affluent suburbs were getting to the hospital. This is an exceptional example, more easily illustrated because of the storm, but these kinds of interpretations are present and these decisions are being made, at least at the bottom end of the medical care system. We need some guidelines because we are making bad decisions, and I'm afraid that a lot of people do place social values on patients.

Prof. Robertson: At other times, decisions have been made on IQ level or perhaps, as in the past, on sex or race. We don't need to get too moralistic about this, but the specter lurking here is a certain arbitrariness in the criteria used. The challenge is to guard against any arbitrariness that clashes with the basic norms that we all honor.

Dr. Mitchell T. Rabkin (General Director, Beth Israel Hospital, Boston): It seems that Prof. Robertson is asking for us to know the unknowable, and Dr. Roe is saying essentially the same thing. Criteria do have to be set, and someday, I hope, they will be, but the point is that decisions have to be made now. In the absence of substantive criteria for who shall live and who shall die, because we don't know how to create them, we ought to pay more attention to the issues of process, which Prof. Robertson spoke about. Those processes, I believe, we can create, and we can develop some consensus on them. For example, think about the difference between physicians assuming full responsibility for decisions made *in camera*, as Dr. Roe suggests, and physicians making physiological judgments and airing the issues openly with all the other caregivers, as described by Prof. Murphy. Documenting the results of these discussions in the medical record, whether the criteria are right or wrong, at least delineates the issues and sets them down for others to see. That is the first step toward this kind of decision making. I would then focus on procedural issues, because the substantive issues are beyond our ken.

Dr. Roe: I don't have any particular difficulty in recognizing such decisions, and my recommendation that guidelines be provided is only to keep me out of jail. It's easy for me, having had to deal rather extensively with these decisions for 35 years. I'm fairly confident in what I'm doing, but I'm sure that lots of people might criticize my individual judgments and might be a good deal less comfortable about making decisions like that. Therefore, society in its present structure requires that we have some basis on which we can make these difficult decisions and be supported in them.

Dr. Todres: Let me add to Dr. Rabkin's remarks about a procedural approach to decision making. Decision making involves an equation into which you put a lot of factors and come up with an answer. Now, our answers today may not be very different from what we came up with in the past, but we have actually added a lot of things to the equation, partly as a result of debates and conferences like this, as well as court cases. Airing these issues has made us more aware of all the various people who can add to this equation, ensuring that everyone who should participate does so. With full participation, we come out with an answer that is really the best we can do under the circumstances, and that's honestly all we can do.

Prof. Robertson: I think you're right, Dr. Rabkin. I would like to know the unknowable, and I'm probably not going to learn very much of it. But with regard to substantive criteria, I believe that they do exist and that we can agree on most of them. For example, if a patient is competent, the patient can decide what happens; if the patient is incompetent, we generally do what serves the interests of the patient to the extent that we can identify those interests. It's only in some extreme cases that it becomes more difficult to identify what the outcome of broadly accepted principles would be. On the whole, I think we have a set of moral precepts that guide us. What remains, perhaps, is to lay them out in such a way that their application in a given case will be clear.

Also, Dr. Rabkin's comment about process is excellent. That's what John Rawls calls pure procedural justice, in that, if we have a good process, then whatever comes out of it is just and fair regardless of the substantive criteria used. In the absence of substantive criteria, I would agree that that is an excellent way to proceed.

Dr. Rabkin: We are not disagreeing, but your point about competence illustrates quite clearly what I mean. I do not think it is possible to set down criteria that will be unequivocally applicable to deciding whether a patient is competent or not. That is, can we put the authority for the decision to live or not in the hands of this particular individual? I don't think we can do it, and I don't think it will work. My focus, then, on the process is to delineate the guidelines as well as possible. Then we can assemble the caregivers and perhaps some outside people and ask how well the patient fulfills the criteria of competence, to whatever extent we have defined it. Having debated the case and come to some consensus, which always opts in the patient's favor, we set it down so that anyone else can see what we knew, what we thought, what we said, and what we did. The decision will have been arrived at openly and displayed openly. That's the important part of the procedural aspect, I believe, because it catches the nooks and crannies of the unknowable part.

Prof. Robertson: Perhaps more cases seem clear to me than to you, but, obviously, there are a lot of unclear cases for which we would have to rely on such a process.

Mr. R. John Wuesthoff (Attorney, Portland, Me.): Perhaps I have misinterpreted some of the comments made by the panelists, but I note an air of fatalism in regard to the ability to give a high standard of care. There has been mention of a limited number of physicians and possibly a limited amount of facilities. If when we talk about social costs we are really talking about economic costs, then we should face that, and that is where fatalism seems to permeate the discussion. We are able to have Marshall Plans in Europe, to send weapons all over the world, to supply everybody with the best foods, and to give the highway lobby the best highways. If the populists can go anywhere and do anything that they want, why can't we use these enormous resources to give the best medical care to everyone?

Prof. Swazey: Having entered ethics from other arenas, I tend to operate out of a practical base of reality, and I think there is a bottom to the barrel; we don't have unlimited resources. Also, I would very much question the assumption that using all our medical technological capabilities to the maximum means that we are necessarily providing the best possible care. Dr. Roe made that point, and I quite agree with it. Many nontreatment decisions are made on the basis of what society does provide, much as we wish it provided more. Most of us would probably agree that institutions for seriously handicapped children are less than desirable. Some nontreatment decisions are made on the basis that it is better for this infant to be dead than to live in a warehouse. That is a value judgment, and it is made as a result of societal judgments of what we want to do for handicapped individuals. If we changed our social priorities, we might well come up with different value decisions. I still question, however, the assumption that providing all possible medical care necessarily makes for the best treatment in all cases.

Ms. Marjorie W. Burke (Attorney, The Carney Hospital, Boston): You said that a societal judgment has been made that it is better for a child not to live than to be put in one of society's warehouses. Speaking through the courts, society at present has not made such a decision. I have been uncomfortable throughout this discussion. I don't know much about the practical treatment of newborns, but certainly in the *McNulty* case[1] the court said that, in society's eyes, it was better for the child to live than to die, even if it was in a warehouse.

Prof. Swazey: I agree that it has not been a societal judgment as the courts would look at it, but rather a societal judgment as interpreted in individual cases by physicians and families, who have often thought it better for the infant to die.

Dr. Todres: As I understand the legal situation concerning defective newborns, parents do not have the right to want a child dead; if that is how they feel, the child can become a ward of the state and the state then has the responsibility. All I can say is that in working with critically ill newborns, in the center of the arena so to speak, I often hear parents voice concern about a child who might survive and require institutionalization; many of these places are very grim. Thus, some parents find it preferable for the child to succumb to the illness, rather than for the child to be supported heroically, to continue suffering, and to survive in an institution that is less than optimal.

I would also like to amplify the *Maine Medical Center* v. *Houle* case. This child had severe cosmetic defects, including maldevelopment of one side of the face and only a single eye; she also had a tracheoesophogeal fistula, which is a connection between the gullet and the windpipe that can be lethal if not tied off. Very competent surgeons were available in Maine to perform the necessary surgery. The pediatrician who first saw the child, and I have spoken with him, believed that her defects were largely cosmetic and that otherwise she was mentally intact; the surgical procedure could be lifesaving, and she subsequently could possibly live a reasonable life with some correction of the cosmetic defects. In court, the judge ruled that the parents did not have the right to make a nontreatment decision for the child and that the child deserved the operative procedure. Subsequently, before the operation was actually carried out, the child had an asphyxial episode, a period in which there was a severe lack of oxygen to the brain, which is very damaging. Now the pediatrician was in a very awkward position. He no longer felt he should perform heroics, but his hands were tied, having already gone to court, and he had to go ahead with the surgery. He had actually changed his viewpoint, which was initially based on a child who would be reasonably intact. If the new situation had prevailed originally, he would not have gone to court.

Prof. Robertson: While there may well be cases where it is in the interest of the child to die rather than to receive medical care, we must be very careful to define the circumstances in which they occur. One perhaps could be that the child was in incessant pain, such that in no way could continued life be conceived of as a benefit. Another case might be that there is no ability to relate to anyone else on any level. But short of such extreme cases, it is very difficult to justify nontreatment of defective newborns on the grounds that it is in their interest. It may not be in the interest of the family, society, the hospital, and others to treat these children, but if that is the case, the decision should be made on those grounds. To say that it is better not to treat this infant so that the child will not have to live in an institution for the rest of life often masks the real judgment that is being made, which is to promote the interest of the parents and maybe society, rather than the child.

Dr. Roe: I sense an inconsistency or a hypocrisy in this discussion. We are dwelling on the importance of involving the patient and the family in these decisions, and we are dealing only with decisions that have to do with the fringe, the end of life or its continuation. Supposedly, we are practicing in a country where there is free choice of medical care; supposedly, we have informed consent, where we go through the charade of signing lots of papers and doing lots of talking. Yet, in my practical experience, very few people ever ask any of the pertinent questions. Physicians decide when someone needs an operation, and physicians call in the surgeons. They never ask patients whether they have a surgeon in mind, whether they even like the surgeon chosen or would prefer to see another one. So the operation is scheduled and performed, and the patient and family just sort of nod their heads and say, "Yes, if that's what you think, sure." We have all sorts of fancy diplomas on our walls that indicate that we are accredited and trained and qualified to do this kind of work, but nobody has ever asked me whether I'm certified by the board. Nobody has ever asked how many times I have done the procedure that I have just recommended or what kind of results I have had. Perhaps, in my three decades of practice, a few have asked, but they are a precious few. From a practical standpoint, the public and the average patient, including intelligent educated ones, simply accept what the doctor recommends. So, why all of a sudden are we making such a big thing about these decisions at one end of the scale when we are not making them in the middle?

Prof. Swazey: The issues of who makes decisions and on what bases, which now figure so prominently in the case of a terminally or critically ill patient, eventually start to generalize down to the more common range of everyday practice. We've seen that happen, for example, with informed consent; it began with human experimentation and moved into medical treatment more generally. I would thus expect that the types of issues we are dealing with today will flow into the less dramatic realms of medical practice.

Dr. Lothar Gidro-Frank (Psychiatrist, Columbia Presbyterian Hospital, New York): It's not hypocrisy that I'm responding to, but a kind of denial of reality that I seem to be hearing. A great deal has been said about the patient's right to make decisions. However, watching what actually happens, as both a physician and a patient, it is much more typical that as soon as patients enter a hospital, they are put on a conveyor belt and cannot get off. There is no way of making decisions from the conveyor belt.

Prof. Swazey: An entire conference could be held on what really happens to patients once they have put on their one-piece open-backed johnny gowns, which are not designed to enable someone to exercise much autonomy, and indeed, patients on that conveyor belt aren't in a very good position to exercise judgment about anything. But to say that is the way the system is should not preclude discussions such as we are having. The next set of questions, then, is should we change the system, and how do we go about it?

Ms. Cynthia Jorgensen (Student, Boston University): If we are aware of resources being scarce, why can't we focus on correcting the problem rather than on developing criteria to decide how to allot those resources? A recent survey indicated that a majority of Americans would be willing to pay more taxes if they knew that the money would go for health care.

Prof. Robertson: The solution is not to pour in more money, because at some point, scarcity simply exists; it's almost a basic law of the universe. Somewhere along the line, decisions have to be made about the allocation of funds and resources.

Dr. Roe: Along with scarcity, we simultaneously have a skyrocketing curve of increased technology. I alluded in my talk to the fact that it is not inconceivable that we could have $100,000 machines that could keep everybody alive indefinitely. That's exaggerated, perhaps, but we are approaching that sort of thing. Do we want to keep everybody alive forever at infinite cost?

Prof. Swazey: There is a difference between allocating resources to correct problems of access to equitable primary care and allocating them so that everybody ends up, as some patients already have, on dialysis machines, with pacemakers, total parenteral nutrition, and a whole range of other medical technologies that essentially keep them alive only biologically. There are various types of allocation decisions and related issues, and morally, we might come out with very different decisions on how we want to allocate resources to areas like primary care or artificial hearts.

Dr. Prout: We are in an era where we are willing to allocate resources, and we do get choosy some days. My basic objection to a utilitarian value-judgment approach to deciding applications of therapy, rather than setting standards for its application, is that the track record of medicine shows that such decisions have not been made solely on physiological grounds but often on the bases of social values. I am especially concerned with that approach because I work with the people who would flunk out.

NOTE

1.   The *McNulty* case, brought before the Massachusetts probate court in the wake of *Saikewicz*, involved an infant whose mother had contracted German measles early in her pregnancy. The infant's early complications included respiratory distress and a heart defect, and according to her physicians, if she survived, she would "probably" be deaf, blind, and severely retarded. The physicians' and parents' joint request to the court for permission not to correct the heart defect was denied under *Saikewicz*, and the surgery was performed.—Eds.

PERSPECTIVES ON DECISION-MAKING PROCEDURES

III

A Physician's Perspective on the *Dinnerstein* Case

Russell J. Rowell, M.D.   **11**

The Massachusetts Appeals Court has approved the use of no-code or do not resuscitate orders without prior judicial approval in certain cases of terminally ill patients. For Massachusetts physicians, the decision *In the Matter of Shirley Dinnerstein* was of great significance because it verified a previous decision of the state's Supreme Judicial Court, which had been interpreted to require unstinting efforts, treatment, and resuscitation of all patients unless a court had authorized a lesser degree of effort in the particular case. This decision, of course, is the *Saikewicz* case, which was handed down in November 1977 and has been talked about ever since. The *Dinnerstein* case was decided by the appeals court, which is the state's second highest tribunal, and the decision is binding because it has not been appealed. While the ruling sanctions the use of no-code orders, it also leaves open the possibility that the attending physician might be sued for malpractice if a no-code order is entered in a negligent way; this, however, seems to be quite a remote possibility.

The *Dinnerstein* case concerned a 67-year-old widow with Alzheimer's disease, which, as far as is known, is incurable. She had had the disease for about six years when her case came to court, and during that time she had also suffered a massive stroke that had left her totally paralyzed on the left side. She was confined to a hospital bed in a vegetative state and required nasogastric feeding, catheterization, and all kinds of maintenance care. Her high blood pressure was complicated by kidney disease as a result of a constricted artery leading to her kidney. Additionally, she had coronary artery disease associated with arteriosclerosis. Although there was no way of knowing when she would die, her life expectancy was thought to be less than a year.

In view of all these facts, the attending physician recommended that in the event of a cardiac or respiratory arrest, resuscitation should not be attempted. The patient's family, including a daughter and a son who was also a physician, agreed with that recommendation. The family, joined by the doctor and the hospital, sought a determination from the probate court as to whether a no-code order could be entered for the patient. The court appointed a guardian ad litem, who posed the request of the physician, and the case was referred to the appeals court.

The case was brought to court in apparent response to the *Saikewicz* decision, in which the Supreme Judicial Court had said that it was the responsibility of the courts to decide whether a seriously ill 67-year-old incompetent person should be treated with a painful but potentially life-prolonging procedure. Invoking the substituted-judgment doctrine, the court made the choice it believed Mr. Saikewicz would have made if he were competent to do so and ruled that the treatment need not be administered. The reasoning was that the treatment was so painful and had such serious side effects that it was likely that competent persons faced with the same choice might refuse treatment; in addition, the form of leukemia that Mr. Saikewicz had would lead to a painless death within a few months.

Despite the high court's ruling that the treatment need not be administered, the *Saikewicz* opinion was taken by the medical profession in Massachusetts to mean that only the judiciary could make the decision to withhold potentially lifesaving or life-prolonging treatment from incompetent terminally ill patients. This led to extraordinary turbulence in the medical community. Physicians wondered whether they had to seek court approval before entering a no-code order or disconnecting a respirator from a terminally ill incompetent patient.

Thus, the need for a case like *Dinnerstein* arose from the uncertainty created by *Saikewicz*. *Dinnerstein* did two things for physicians. It clarified the fact that *Saikewicz* did not require prior court approval for all decisions not to treat incompetent terminally ill patients, and it set up specific circumstances under which prior approval is not necessary. The case thus creates a separate category of terminally ill patients who, as far as the court in Massachusetts is concerned, do not need to be resuscitated in the event of cardiac or respiratory arrest. For this group of patients, the decision not to resuscitate is up to the physician and the family. This category comprises patients who cannot by any means be cured of their underlying terminal disease and for whom death is near. While the appeals court did not say how near death must be, a reasonable inference from *Dinnerstein* would be within one year, because the life expectancy of Mrs. Dinnerstein was a year or less.

Perhaps the most striking aspect of the court's opinion is its discussion of the phenomenon of dying. The court pointed out that death is not only a state, but also a process with which physicians are not obliged to interfere. In concluding that no-code orders may be entered under such circumstances as described, the court stated that cessation of heartbeat and respiration is part of the normal process of dying and, as such, does not represent a condition for which medical treatment should be required as a matter of law. The court noted that the extreme reading of *Saikewicz* would require attempts to resuscitate dying patients with cardiac or respiratory arrest in a manner that could be characterized as a pointless, even cruel, prolongation of the act of dying.

Although a traditional concept of the physician's duty has been to prolong life, it is apparent that in a case such as *Dinnerstein*, some consideration must be given to the kind of life that is being prolonged. For Mrs. Dinnerstein, who suffered from progressive brain disease, life following a successful resuscitation effort could never be anything but a continued lingering in a vegetative state. For her, prolongation of life would be, in the court's phrase, a mere suspension of the act of dying. The type of life that the *Dinnerstein* court believed the *Saikewicz* decision was intended to preserve is the normal, functioning, integrative existence of healthy human beings, and not a continued lingering in a vegetative state.

Present in both this and the *Saikewicz* case was the incompetence of the patient. While in *Saikewicz* the court was willing to step in to make the choice that the patient would make if he were competent, the *Dinnerstein* court said that it need not act to make the choice for the patient because, in that situation, there was really no choice to be made. Because *Dinnerstein* does not distinguish between patients who are competent and those who are not, it brings up some new legal problems. In either event, the court stated, the decision regarding a no-code order should be made by the physician. Attempts to apply resuscitation in cases such as *Dinnerstein*, if successful, will do nothing to cure or relieve the illness that brought the patient to the threshold of death. The case does not, therefore, present the type of significant treatment choice that, in the light of sound medical advice, is to be made by the patient if competent to do so. Since *Dinnerstein* does not present the possibility of lifesaving or life-prolonging treatment described in *Saikewicz*, the decision does not turn on the patient's competence or lack of it. Instead, *Dinnerstein* involves a question relating to the process of death itself, and on that basis, the court was willing to place the responsibility for the decision on the physician.

The court felt that, once the process of death begins, it is up to the medical profession to decide how to ease the passing of an irreversibly terminally ill patient in light of the patient's history and condition and the wishes of the family. The question is not one for judicial decision, but rather for the attending physician, in keeping with the highest traditions of the medical profession. It is subject to court review only to the extent that it may be contended that the physician had not exerted the degree of care and skill of the average qualified practitioner, taking into account advances in the profession. The court is apparently saying that a physician who issues a no-code order may be subject to medical malpractice liability if the order is entered negligently but will not be subject to any other liability, civil or criminal.

As helpful as the *Dinnerstein* case is in clearing up some of the problems physicians face with terminal patients, the decision does not answer a number of quesions. For example, in that case, the patient's life expectancy was a year or less. What happens when the life expectancy is not known? What if a patient is in a vegetative, irreversible condition but might live for two years? What if a member of the patient's family protests a no-code order on the grounds—unrealistic as they may be—that a cure may be found if the patient is kept alive? What if a patient is so brain damaged as to be helpless but is not suffering from a terminal illness? And finally, does *Dinnerstein* authorize disconnection of an artificial life-support system under circumstances in which it would approve entry of a no-code order? Answers to these questions, and many others, must await formal consideration of actual cases.

The greatest contribution of *Dinnerstein* is the evidence it provides that the Massachusetts judiciary is willing to be realistic about the problems of dealing with dying patients. No one denies that no-code orders have been issued and followed for some time; this fact was acknowledged recently by the New Jersey Supreme Court in the *Quinlan* case. Now for the first time, Massachusetts physicians may be secure about issuing no-code orders within the limits of *Dinnerstein*. To require the kind of court proceedings that *Saikewicz* seemed to require only increases the burden, during an already difficult time, for both the family and the physician. Whether or not such requirements are followed, their mere presence at a time of stress serves to create resentment. In cases like *Dinnerstein*, where no real choice exists, mandating that a court charade be acted out, with no effect on the patient's condition, only creates disrespect for the law. It is to be hoped that other states will follow Massachusetts's lead.

Advocacy:
An Ethical Model
for Assisting Patients
with Treatment Decisions

Sally Gadow, R.N., Ph.D.   **12**

The concept was introduced earlier of the professional person who is philosophically in charge of a case or a patient. I want to direct my remarks to a belief that seemed to underlie a great many of the subsequent comments, which is that it is the patient who is philosophically in charge, whenever possible, rather than a professional.

As difficult as decision making is for nonparticipating patients, it is at least equally difficult with regard to patients who are able to decide. That is the difficulty I shall address—namely, the need for a procedure for patients to follow in decision making or, more to the point, for health professionals to follow in assisting patients in the process of decision making.

On the one hand, we may be reluctant to grant that such decisions are rightfully the patients', and on the other, we are often relieved when decision making has been established to be "the patient's problem." These two different feelings reflect two different models for procedure making, and I shall propose a third model.

The first model is the familiar stance of paternalism, which assumes that individuals ought to be urged, if not forced, to select treatment or nontreatment according to what the professionals consider to be in the patients' best interests. In this model, for example, the role of the nurse as the physician's accomplice might be to engineer the consent of a patient to a course of action that is expressly not desired by that individual. Nurses often exercise great and subtle powers, and therefore such a procedure for decision making is entirely feasible.

The extreme of the paternalistic model is the "grateful relief syndrome," which I shall refer to as the consumerism model. Here, there is no desire by the professionals to shoulder the decision-making burden; rather, they are thankful that the patients' rights movement has relocated the problem to the patient's domain. In this model, the nurse is a consumer advocate who supplies the patient with all the facts of the case and then discretely withdraws, leaving the decision entirely in the hands of the so-called consumer. Notice that the withdrawal of the professional is as vital to the procedure as the providing of information, since this model assumes that a patient might be unduly influenced by so much as a frown or a sigh if the decision is not made in the strictest privacy. At most, a professional, highly skilled in noncommunication, might provide a listening ear while the patient deliberates out loud.

Both models, though perhaps appealing for their own reasons, fail to address the problem that I proposed—the need for a procedure to assist patients in decision making. Paternalism regards patients as temporarily incompetent; there is, therefore, no possibility of their making a decision, either with or without assistance. Consumerism regards patients as partially nonhuman, a computer requiring nothing more than appropriate input in order to process a decision; there is no need of assistance beyond purely technical aid. Thus, we see that one of these procedures dispenses with the patient and the other dispenses with the professional. In neither case does the professional assist the patient in the decision process itself.

I propose a third model, which will accomplish just that. I call it the advocacy model. Despite the lure of paternalism and consumerism, I believe that advocacy ought to be the ethical model for professionals in patient decision making.

A word of caution, first. Advocacy is understood in some contexts to mean acting on behalf of someone. While that meaning is important in certain circumstances, it is the opposite of what I have in mind. In my model, advocacy means assisting patients in their own actions, rather than substituting professional actions and decisions for those of patients. The view of advocacy as decision making on behalf of patients, in fact, approaches the paternalistic model, whereas the view I am suggesting provides a clear alternative to paternalism and consumerism.

Specifically, advocacy is actively assisting patients in their free self-determination of treatment options. Advocacy not only safeguards but also positively contributes to the exercise of self-determination. In concrete terms, it is an effort to help individuals become clear about what they want in a situation, to assist them in discerning and clarifying their values, and to help them in examining available options in light of their values. This assistance takes place in the form of discussions between the professional and the patient. Among the purposes of these discussions that are mutually agreed upon by professionals and patients is the clarification of the patients' values, including, in the case of nontreatment decisions, the views of dying and death that these individuals hold or would like to hold.

The suggestion that advocacy ought to be the ethical model for assisting patients in decision making assumes two things: that such assistance is needed and that it is possible. In considering the first assumption, it would seem that at no time is the need to clarify someone's values more urgent than in deciding on measures that will affect the quality and, indeed, the continuation of that person's life. Yet at the very time that such deliberation is the most needed, it is frequently the most difficult. The values and beliefs that are called into question in such circumstances are often those that are the most deeply imbedded and unquestioned in a person's life, as well as perhaps the least defined and developed. This first assumption, that is, the need for assistance, sets the advocacy model clearly apart from consumerism, which assumes a need only for information. The second assumption distinguishes advocacy from paternalism because it assumes that such assistance is possible—that is, patients can be helped noncoercively to reach decisions.

If advocacy, then, is both necessary and possible, how do we go about it? I believe that the advocacy model suggests a procedure, or at least guidelines, for assisting patients with treatment decisions. Several distinct considerations need to be addressed by nurses and other professionals practicing advocacy, considerations that derive from the concept of advocacy itself. The conceptual themes, or components, of advocacy that I will identify here are: (1) self-determination, (2) the patient-practitioner relationship, (3) the practitioner's values, (4) the patient's values, and (5) individuality. If we think of the ideal of advocacy as a thread running through a person's professional practice, these five themes would then be the strands within that thread; and for the ideal to be fully realized in a particular situation, all five strands would have to be involved, that is, all five considerations would have to be heeded. Each theme might be seen as a general area for discussion between a patient and a professional. But perhaps more importantly, each must be carefully addressed by professionals in their own ethical reflections throughout the advocacy relationship with patients.

Let me illustrate how these themes can serve as guidelines or as a conceptual procedure for advocacy by discussing them with reference to an imaginary situation. Suppose that a terminally ill woman, who has not been told her prognosis, is contemplating recommended surgical treatment and asks a nurse whether she should undergo the operation.

The first concept, that of self-determination or autonomy, seems to be the central theme. In all cases, but in this one specifically, this concept brings up the matter of information on the basis of which our patient can understand the situation as well as alternative ways of responding to it. In the advocacy model, the more information that is available to our patient, the more informed and thus the more free her decision can be. The choice of surgery versus nonsurgery is not so free a decision as is the choice of surgery over chemotheraphy, radiation, visualization therapy, herbal medicine, or nontreatment. In my model it is not necessary to defend a patient's right to know, because the need for relevant information is presupposed by the concept of self-determination. It would also be inconsistent to fail to provide whatever information the individual requires to exercise self-determination. It would clearly be impossible for the woman to give informed, and therefore free, consent to a surgical procedure if she does not know, for example, that the expected outcome is at most an additional six months of life, especially in view of the fact that she is not aware of her prognosis.

Now a problem arises—does the concept of self-determination, with its requirement for full information, mean that professional assistance amounts to no more than consumer protection, that is, announcement of all the options followed by a hasty retreat? Alternatively, does it mean that patients sometimes ought to have information forced on them that they may not want? With these questions, we are led to the second theme of advocacy, the nature of the relationship between the patient and practitioner. Since the goal of that relationship in the advocacy model is to assist patients in their self-determination, both the paternalistic and the consumerist procedures for providing information are faulty. In fact, they share a common fault; they assume that the amount and type of information that is appropriate can be determined without patient participation. If the selection of information is the decision of the professional, rather than the patient, less or more may be given than is needed, or what is given may be irrelevant from the patient's point of view. Thus, the neutral objectivity of the consumer model is reduced to paternalism because the decision is made for the patient.

Here it would seem that the avenue most consistent with the advocacy relationship between the professional and patient would be to enable—not just allow—the patient to determine the selection of information that is to be presented. In tactical terms, this might be accomplished by either indirect or direct kinds of ways. A direct inquiry might involve the following questions, although not all of them and certainly not all at the same time: "Would you be helped in making your decision if you had more information? If you knew more about the clinical findings? If you knew the expected outcomes of alternatives? If you knew what the prognosis is thought to be? If you knew your family's feelings in the matter? If you knew the views of persons who have faced similar decisions?" A less direct way of inviting a patient to determine the extent of information needed might be for nurses to express their own views. For example, a nurse might say to the patient we discussed earlier, "I think it is helpful if people find out about all the alternatives before making up their minds. Do you feel this way?" In short, advocacy in this situation defines the nurse-patient relationship in terms of assisting this patient not only in deciding about the recommended treatment, but also first in determining the selection of information she wishes to have, assuming, of course, that any information she requests will be given freely.

The theme that emerges now, the third component, is that of the practitioner's values, especially the position of those values in a discussion that has the purpose of promoting the patient's self-determination. I believe that the practitioner's values should be a part of the information to which a patient is entitled. This belief is valid not because of a right of the patient to know these values, but because it is a function of the advocacy relationship itself. To the extent that the patient enters the relationship as a so-called "whole person," the professional, too, must be fully present. This means that, although the patient's values will be decisive, the values of the professional have to be expressed as well. Moreover, it is especially important that they be expressed when they conflict with the patient's.

If we have indeed given up the authoritarian model of health care, there is no reason to suppose that the communication of the practitioner's values is necessarily coercive. On the contrary, such disclosure would seem to serve several purposes. At a minimum, it provides this patient with information that she may find useful in understanding the professional's behavior toward her. But even more, it may offer her an example of an alternative view, one that she might want to take into account in considering her own values. Just as there is no basis outside the authoritarian model for assuming that a patient will capitulate instantly after discovering that the practitioner has a different view, there is likewise no reason for supposing that a patient would never want to consider another's values. Nothing prevents professionals from changing their minds after discussions with patients; similarly, the possibility always exists that the patient might choose to modify her position after reflecting on the nurse's views.

The purpose of the disclosure, of course, is not to persuade the patient, but neither is it merely to give information. It amounts to an affirmation to the patient that the practitioner is concerned with the articulation of values, not as an impersonal prescription for decision making, but as a personal commitment to ethical reflection.

Thus, we see that the ultimate purpose in disclosing the professional's values is to assist clarification of the patient's values, which leads to my fourth conceptual theme. One value that is fundamental in treatment decisions concerns the quality of life that the patient desires or at least deems acceptable. In other words, it must be determined whether a proposed measure will sustain or significantly diminish the quality of life that the patient values. Quality-of-life determinations are usually based on professional notions about the meaning of a life that is characterized by suffering, terminal illness, or continuous treatment. In the advocacy model, however, only the values of the patient concerning the quality of her own life are to be decisive.

Directly related to patient values is the concept of individuality, the final theme of advocacy. In assisting patient decision making, it is important to distinguish individuality from the closely related theme of values, because considerations other than values per se can be decisive in a patient's self-determination. I group these last considerations under the concept of individuality. Persons are a composite of their unique understanding and experience of themselves and of their bodies and their relationship between self and body. The unity or disunity between self and body that patients experience can significantly affect their decisions, particularly in a terminal illness when the value of the self-body relationship itself may be in question. We see this occasionally in persons who perceptually or emotionally negate the reality of a body part that is, to them, already dead.

Thus, advocacy in the situation here would involve assistance to this patient in ascertaining the way in which she experiences her body. She might perceive it as only a shell for her soul, a shell that can be relinquished relatively easily if she believes that the soul lives after her body's death. Or she may experience the unity of self and body as utterly indissoluble, and thus the death of the body would mean the annihilation of her entire being. From the patient's view of her body and its relation to the self arises one of the most crucial aspects of individuality in these kinds of decisions, and that is the patient's personal views concerning death. Here, advocacy involves a unique and distinctly philosophical task. To assist terminally ill persons in their free determination of the way in which they want to understand their dying and death requires a level of participation that penetrates to the heart of existence, uncovering and clarifying fears, longings, hopes, and beliefs, so that an understanding of death can be found or created that expresses the full individuality of that person.

These five conceptual strands within advocacy provide a means of establishing procedures for patient decision making arising out of the model of advocacy. Paternalism and consumerism are other models, and they suggest other procedures. In our concern to formulate professional decision-making procedures for nonparticipating patients, it is imperative that we not overlook the fact that, either consciously or unconsciously, we are simultaneously establishing procedures for dealing with patients who can make their own decisions. My model is an attempt to help us establish these procedures consciously rather than unconsciously.

Immunizing Physicians by Law[1]

Robert A. Burt, J.D.

13

Today, when physicians and patients are trying to decide whether or not to end treatment, the automatic response seems to be to call for a lawyer. I want to address the question of how lawyers became involved in the first place. Let me begin with the time of innocence—before *Saikewicz* and *Quinlan*—and see if we can figure out how we got to this point.

In the old days, if a physician asked a lawyer for a treatment decision like that in *Saikewicz*, the lawyer would reply, "Are you asking me whether you should turn off the respirator or withhold treatment? I am not the one to answer that question. Who else have you talked to? What does the patient say? The family? What about your colleagues and other professionals? What is in the literature about established procedures in this area? And finally—if not first—what do the family and the patient, the people most immediately affected, want to hear?"

Now let us assume that all concerned parties, including a lucid patient, agree to stop the treatment and the doctor wants assurance from the attorney that it is safe to do so. The physician is not satisfied with the attorney saying it sounds like a "good risk"; rather, the doctor is seeking complete assurance against both civil liability and criminal responsibility. Any sensible lawyer would have to reply that it is not possible to give binding and absolute assurance. For example, if an estate administrator brings suit and the patient had signed a piece of paper with a blanket authorization for all kinds of procedures, this paper may not stand up in court. The patient, after all, was in a very necessitous position, and in positions of great inequality of power, courts look very skeptically at waivers of rights. It is unlikely, but conceivable, that the court would hold the physician liable.

It seems to me that physicians should concede that risks are a part of their job and they should feel confident about making decisions without the promise of complete immunity. In fact, however, this is not what has happened in Massachusetts and elsewhere. Increasingly, physicians are unwilling to take any kind of measurable legal risk. They are not used to doing so, and they do not like the possibility that somebody, somewhere, might decide that a decision they made was unjustified.

Why is that so? It has to do, in part, with fears of malpractice suits and the belief that such suits are mushrooming. The fact that the problem appears so acute to physicians in Massachusetts also has to do with the Edelin prosecution, which was unprecedented in its own terms.[2] At the same time, our society seems to be undergoing fundamental changes in attitudes toward authority figures in general and physicians in particular; there appears to be more skepticism, more of a feeling that physicians and professionals have been overreaching their role. Consumers are beginning to assert their prerogatives.

All these factors have left physicians very unsettled. They are no longer willing to take risks because they have lost confidence in their old belief of immunity from liability. It is this unwillingness to take risks that has produced the court interventions that *Saikewicz* represents. This is a very unfortunate attitude, and unless this attitude changes among physicians, we will continue to encounter the kinds of rigidity, awkwardness, hypocrisy, and compounded confusion that have come in the wake of the *Saikewicz* case.

Let me move from the lawyer-doctor relationship to suggest an analogy that I hope will make sense to physicians. Consider a patient suffering from cancer, for example, that is discovered in the early stages and operated on. The patient wants to know whether the physician got it all out and is not satisfied with an answer of "pretty confident"; the patient wants total assurance. When the physician explains that the nature of life and medical practice makes such complete assurance impossible, the patient replies, "I cannot live that way. I must have a sense of complete immunity. I didn't used to be sick and now I want to be completely cured. What can you do?" The physician then discusses the options of chemotherapy, radiation therapy, and further exploratory surgery but adds that they all have serious side effects and that the patient will end up feeling sicker. In other words, the physician advises that the cure is worse than the disease and that the patient would be better off living with some uncertainty. The patient, however, may not be willing to live with this uncertainty and may insist that the physician do absolutely everything possible.

I think that this is what doctors are doing now when they go to court. Lawyers have told physicians that they cannot give 100 percent assurance of legal immunity, that only judges can give this guarantee through the issuance of declaratory judgments. That is, lawyers have correctly advised that the only way physicians can have complete immunity from civil or criminal liability is to go to court before making a treatment decision, present all the facts to the judge, and ask the judge for "the right answer." Increasingly, doctors are replying, "Terrific! That's what I want." But here, too, the cure is worse than the disease.

I believe that it is not good to bring judges into the medical decision-making process in this before-the-fact or declaratory-judgment mode on any kind of regular basis. The process of judicial involvement and deliberation contains an incredible amount of rigidity and artificiality. Although court procedures are set up to further deliberation through testimony, cross examination, and discussion, the mode of deliberation in reality is highly stylized. The result frequently is rigid role playing among the adversaries, which obstructs sensible, free-flow deliberation. Without free-flow deliberation, the essence of the case gets lost.

Quinlan is another example of physicians unwilling to act on their own. One of the critical elements to be decided was whether Ms. Quinlan needed the respirator to survive. Indeed, the lower court's decision rested on the assumption that turning off the respirator would end her life. And yet, three years have gone by since the respirator was turned off. Although the basic assumption was that she needed the respirator, the fact is that she did not.

Was there an error in judgment? Has the fact that she still lives taken everybody by surprise? It has not. At the trial, one of the physicians, Dr. Fred Plum, who is probably the leading expert in this country on vegetative comas, testified that he had examined Ms. Quinlan and had taken her off the respirator for a short period; in his judgment, she did not need the respirator, although he stated that he would like to test this proposition further. His understanding of the physiology of her illness was that her breathing function was not really interfered with. What then happened was that other physicians, who were less experienced, disagreed with Dr. Plum. (That alone, however, is not unusual, since disagreement always enters into complicated matters.)

If this had truly been a sensible decision-making process, once it was recognized that a real medical question existed, the decision makers should have gone to the bedside and tested the question. But that is not the way court deliberations work. Instead, the court moved on to the next witness; nobody stopped to say, "Here is an interesting question, and here is a way to answer it. Let's do it." By then, the record was fixed, and courts typically prefer to deliberate on the basis of fixed records. Consequently, the essence of the case simply was lost. The decision was made as if it were a fictional case, having nothing to do with a real situation. In my view, that happens again and again in a court setting; both the technological reality and, more importantly, the human reality are overlooked.

This leads me to another observation. The type of deliberative process that Prof. Gadow described, although very hard to conceptualize, is a model that I am very sympathetic toward. This interactional model involves the patient and the professionals, as well as all those around the patient, in an effort to help everybody understand what is at stake as the parties sort out facts and feelings over time, as they swing back and forth between more confusion and less confusion. These cases pose incredible moral dilemmas; they are difficult to decide because they are very confusing. If the answers were clear-cut, there would be no need for discussions such as this conference. To me, confusion such as this is called for in these cases; an interactional model over time is necessary. But this is precisely what cannot take place in a courtroom. When you move into the courts, even if the proceedings involve a competent patient who, for example, demands the right to die, everything automatically becomes stylized. Attorneys are present; people stop talking freely or even directly to one another. The process loses sight of the human element, and the case comes across in storybook fashion.

In my judgment, this leads to irresponsible decision making, which is exactly contrary to the expressed purpose of the courts. The *Saikewicz* opinion, for example, recognizes that important values are at stake and that fully responsible treatment decisions must be made. It says that judges alone have the proper authority and the true responsibility in this society to make these kinds of moral decisions. On its face, that is very appealing. But in fact, the dynamics of court intervention merely confuse the lines of responsibility instead of clarifying them.

Let me illustrate this confusion for one aspect of *Saikewicz*. Toward the very end of the hearing, the trial judge said he was inclined to order treatment. This remark occurred immediately after a brief dialogue in which the judge admitted that the case was perplexing and that the responsibility weighed heavily on him. One of the principal physicians agreed that the decision was most difficult, adding something like, "I don't have that kind of deep knowledge. It is your decision, not mine, and I am glad that I don't have to make it." But when the judge suggested that he might order treatment, the two physicians who would conduct the treatment immediately raised several arguments: that Mr. Saikewicz would be hard to treat, that he would struggle and could not cooperate, and in effect, that the physicians simply did not know what to do with him. As a result, the judge changed his mind. Nonetheless, he sought assurance from the hospital lawyer that the lawyer, not the judge, would write the order. Finally, the judge said something like, "With doctors and professionals in attendance, I hereby reach the decision that treatment should not be given." All of this took place in just a few minutes; this exchange comprises only three typewritten pages in the transcript.

The real question is who made the decision, the judge or the doctors? Most likely, each of them went home thankful that someone else had made the decision. And that to me is the heart of the problem. A decision has indeed been made, but everybody pretends that the other guy did it. The pretense takes place in a very comfortable setting, with all the parties recognizing that if they keep the charade going long enough for the judge to issue an order, then nobody involved in the proceedings will suffer adverse consequences; all will be immune. Nobody will suffer, that is, except the patient. Indeed, the patient will suffer no matter what the decision is, for these are complicated and difficult problems. But once again, the patient's suffering becomes lost while everybody else is seeking immunity from suffering. All in the name of protecting patients, we are setting up a procedural format in which some pretty cold-blooded decisions are likely to be made. We have started ourselves on what lawyers call a slippery slope.

There is one more aspect of *Saikewicz* that I find chilling. Mr. Saikewicz would have suffered, I am sure, had he received chemotherapy. Yet, in this country today, as physicians can testify, virtually all mentally competent people with the same kind of leukemia elect to have chemotherapy in the hopes of extending their lives even for six months or a year. Although it may have been cruel to impose that kind of suffering on Mr. Saikewicz, consider what the court did do. The court withheld treatment that might have prolonged the life of a retarded person in the exact situation in which it believed that mentally normal persons would have received treatment. It seems to me that the cold-bloodedness of such a decision can only gather force in the kind of charade that the judiciary offers. It is a frightening prospect, but the likelihood exists of moving from a retarded person with a terminal illness to retarded or senile old people in general to anomalous newborns. We are proceeding in this direction without realizing it. And we are doing so because the people involved with these troublesome patients want immunity.

What I think the law should embrace is not the withholding of treatment from incompetent patients but the withholding of immunity from those who seek it. The law should not give physicians absolute certainty that they will not be sued. Physicians must be willing to assume some significant risk of adverse results, if only to force them to empathize with the patient, who is also in the midst of a dilemma.

This will not result in tidy solutions to the problem. Indeed, it is the antithesis of drawing up a complete code, such as the court seemed to offer in *Saikewicz*, in which doctors have only to look up the answer as in a cookbook. It is not possible to formulate answers such as, "If the patient's life expectancy is only a year, the respirator can be turned off, but not if the life expectancy is two years; or if the patient is 73, treatment can be withheld, but 42 is a different story." *Saikewicz* seems to imply this kind of code, and I am afraid that physicians are going to be asking the same kind of help from legislators, who may be tempted to formulate such codes. I believe that this is precisely the wrong way to proceed. If we want to preserve our humanity in this process, we must make absolutely certain that we do not end up doing terrible, cruel things in the name of kindness and responsibility.

NOTES

1. Adapted from R. A. Burt. *Taking care of strangers: the rule of law in doctor-patient relations.* New York: The Free Press, 1979.

2. In April 1974, Dr. Kenneth Edelin, then the chief resident of obstetrics and gynecology at Boston City Hospital, was indicted for manslaughter in connection with a legal abortion performed at the hospital in October 1973. In a widely publicized and controversial trial, Dr. Edelin was convicted of manslaughter in the death of a "baby boy." His February 1975 conviction was subsequently overturned by the Massachusetts Supreme Judicial Court. — Eds.

Learning to Live with Judges [1]

George J. Annas, J.D., M.P.H. **14**

Elisabeth Kübler-Ross recounts five stages of reactions to dying that, she holds, every patient goes through: denial, anger, bargaining, depression, and acceptance. Medical professionals in Massachusetts have gone through at least four of these stages since the *Saikewicz* case. They went through denial, originally saying that nothing had changed and therefore they did not have to worry about the case. Then they became angry as they learned more about the opinion and felt that judges were stepping into their territory. Next, the medical community started bargaining with the legislature, saying "Can't we pass a statute to reverse this case?" Many of them are now in the depression stage, as revealed in comments like "This is just awful. The judges are now involved, but we can't do anything about it." It is my hope that the acceptance stage will finally be reached, but I am not sure that I agree with Prof. Burt that we have to accept complete uncertainty.

I am going to discuss a schematic for decision making at different times for patients. The first breakdown is between decisions involving competent patients and those involving incompetent patients, a very primary distinction. Decisions are further subdivided according to the criteria on which they are being made:

medical, legal, or personal. We can obviously argue about the difference between legal and personal criteria, and the divisions are presented not as definitive but only to provoke thought and discussion.

As Prof. Glantz stated so well in his presentation, a competent patient essentially has the legal right to refuse treatment for any reason and, I would argue, for absolutely any reason. In *Quinlan* and *Saikewicz*, we have two cases in which state supreme courts have said that, under certain circumstances, there may be some compelling state interests that might permit the state to step into the case. These interests are the value of life, the prevention of suicide, the protection of innocent third parties such as children, and the maintenance of the ethical integrity of the medical profession. But both courts made it very clear that none of these state interests applies to a terminally ill competent patient; there are simply no circumstances under which a court can override a competent, terminally ill patient's desire not to be treated.

That is all I want to say about competent patients, because I do not think they constitute the major problem, although they do represent an extremely important one. The *Quinlan* and *Saikewicz* cases make their rights clear, and these are the first state supreme court cases to do so. Indeed, they are the first state supreme court cases, subsequent to the U.S. Supreme Court's abortion decision enunciating the right to privacy, to talk about refusing treatment. The most important thing about these two decisions is that they clarified for the first time the constitutional rights of competent patients. What they did not make clear, however, are the rights of incompetent patients.

Turning now to incompetent patients, the first set of criteria on which we might make a decision not to treat is medical. Three primary medical criteria have been recognized by the courts, the first being death. Doctors are the ones who declare someone is dead, and when someone is dead, that person does not have to be treated. That does not sound terribly controversial to me, but cases involving some people who are brain dead have been brought to court in Massachusetts since *Saikewicz*, and the judge has been asked, "Do we have to treat these corpses?" The answer is obviously "no" and should not require judicial sanction.

The second criterion is a little more nebulous, but it has been consistently upheld by the courts; physicians do not have to treat a "hopeless" patient. Almost by definition, nothing can be done for a hopeless person. Much can be done *to* a hopeless person, but treatment is not required, for there is no therapy that will work. Who decides when someone is hopeless? Medical professionals make this decision, and they do so based on "good and accepted medical practice." I do not believe that physicians should ever want the courts to become any more specific than that. It is silly, for example, to say that with 1-year life expectancy, we will keep someone on a respirator, but with 11 months, we will turn it off. That kind of certainty will never come from a court (or a physician), nor should anyone ask for or expect it. "Hopeless," I think, is the right type of criterion, the meaning of which is supplied by current technology and practice.

The *Quinlan* court went one step further, following testimony by physicians that "We can never say never." There are always miracles, and the physicians would not say that it was impossible for Ms. Quinlan to recover. Thus, the *Quinlan* criterion is that treatment can be discontinued if there is "no reasonable possibility of the patient returning to a cognitive, sapient state." This criterion has been accepted in New Jersey, and if the medical community adopted it as a standard, it would probably be accepted by courts in other states as well.

I call these three criteria "medical" because I contend that they are decisions that doctors can make themselves on the basis of their own expertise. They do not have to go to the family and say, "Your husband is dead; may we take him off the respirator?" That makes no sense, even though that is the law in North Carolina. There are certain things that we as a society have said physicians are capable of doing and competent to do, and we rely on physicians to do them. The courts have specifically stated that these three examples are properly within medical authority.[2]

Probably the main reason that the *Quinlan* case was brought to court was that the medical malpractice "crisis" was at its height. We were aware of scare tactics. For example, let me quote what the president of the State Trial Lawyers Association said in New York in 1975: "People in high positions in the medical profession are trying to create a crisis so they can abolish malpractice suits and then they can kill anybody they want to and it will not make any difference." *Medical Economics* suggested that doctors had better watch out for lawyers because "the malpractice hustlers are on the prowl." Lawyers were portrayed as wolves in sheep's clothing. Thus, there was some justification for the doctors in the *Quinlan* case to say that, given this kind of atmosphere, they were not going to do anything in the public light unless the court said it was all right.

Therefore, the Quinlan physicians went to court. And they did so, I believe, to ask three questions that the courts are set up to answer: Is what we want to do classifiable as murder? Is it negligence? Is it fair and reasonable? The last question is a different kind of test. Homicide and negligence are areas that courts deal with frequently, although they usually do so after the fact. They say, for example, that what John Jones did is murder in the first degree or the second degree, or it was malpractice, and they decide to send the case to the jury. No one else can make these decisions, and absolutely no one else in our society has the mandate to make them.

Lawyers can give advice and often do give advice with 99 percent certainty. But no one except a court can give 100 percent certainty and a guarantee of immunity. The only place to get this type of legal immunity is in a court. That is perfectly appropriate, and I do not see why anyone would want anyone else to be able to grant legal immunity. Even the *Quinlan* court retained to itself the power to give immunity; it did not delegate ultimate authority to an ethics committee except when very narrow and explicit criteria could be applied.

The third question, as to whether something is fair and reasonable, argues that we go to court not so much because the court can make the decision, but because the court represents the public morals and thus should have a chance to tell physicians whether what they are planning to do is "fair and reasonable." It is, for example, the criterion applied to some bone-marrow transplant cases involving minor donors. Physicians do not take bone-marrow transplant cases to court to find out whether it is criminal or constitutes malpractice; they go to court to see whether it is fair and reasonable, that is, to protect the donor against possible conflicts of interest on the part of the parents.

Finally, and by far the most difficult, are what I call "personal" criteria, although both the *Quinlan* and the *Saikewicz* courts categorized them as "legal." They are the other reasons why a decision might be made not to treat an incompetent patient. One is the belief that it is in the person's best interests—that is, the person might be better off—not to be treated. The second is the belief that if the person were competent to make a decision, the person would say, "Do not treat me."

The best interests test is a strange kind of test. It is a traditional legal test, for example, in custody cases, in which everybody always tries to do what is in the best interests of the child. Whenever children are before the courts, there will usually be a best interests test, and guardians are supposed to do what is best for their wards.

The question that immediately comes to mind, and has certainly come to the mind of many physicians, is "Why are courts better at this than doctors?" This is followed by a second question, "Is this the kind of thing courts usually do?" The answer to this question is "no." Courts usually examine past events, as when a trial is held after an automobile accident to determine who was at fault, who caused the accident, and who should pay how much. Or who is guilty of a rape or a murder. Or what the legal status is of the parties involved. When courts look at past events, they are looking at something that is not in itself going to be affected by what they decide. The court system has proved very good at trying to figure out what has happened and at sorting out liabilities for past events.

This is, however, completely different from what the courts are being asked to do in a *Saikewicz* or a *Quinlan* type of case. They are not being asked to determine what happened in the past, but rather what we should do in the future to a specific person. What kind of decision should we make to ensure that this person's best interests are going to be protected? Some legal literature suggests that the courts are not very good at making this type of decision in an area such as child custody cases.[3] The decision usually ends up serving the best interests of one or both parents rather than the child. Courts do not know any more about the best interests of children than do social workers, other people professionally involved, or parents. They cannot predict the future any better than you or I can or any better than psychiatrists can predict dangerousness (much legal literature exists on how difficult the concept of dangerousness has been for the courts).

Another reason why the best interests test might not be suitable for judicial determination is that, since it is so individualized, it has very limited precedential value; and one purpose for going to court is to set a precedent so that further court cases along the same lines may not be necessary. In other words, a court may say, "If this circumstance holds, do this." However, when a decision is based on the best interests of a particular child, that child is different from any other child, and one ward is different from any other ward. Had *Saikewicz* been decided by using the best interests test, the fact that Mr. Saikewicz was not treated certainly would not mean that mentally retarded people no longer have to be treated for cancer. It would mean only that the court, under those circumstances and in that particular case, found that it was in the best interests of Mr. Saikewicz not to be treated. Now, if another person came along with substantially identical circumstances, it would still be necessary to go to court under the best interests test to seek another determination as to what is in the best interests of that particular person, because that person would not be Mr. Saikewicz.

Thus, it seems clear that problems exist in using the best interests test in court. In this regard, I am sympathetic to the claim of many physicians, which is that physicians are in a better position than judges to determine what is in their patients' best interests. To a point, this is true. Physicians obviously know more than judges do about their patients' families, the patients' circumstances, and of course, their diseases. If we simply substitute judicial paternalism for medical paternalism, we achieve nothing. That clearly does not help patients. I am not arguing that medical paternalism is good, but rather that judicial paternalism is probably no better.

A corollary is that it is inappropriate for judges to go to a patient's bedside to view the extent of the illness or injury, if their decision is going to be influenced by how sick the person looks or what the probability is of the person's getting better. Those judgments are medical decisions. Probably the only time judges should go to a patient's bedside is when they need to decide whether the patient is competent or incompetent. Judges may then want to find out for themselves whether the patient can understand the nature of the disease and its probable course with and without treatment. In those circumstances, I agree that judges should go to the patient's bedside. But to do so under other circumstances smacks of "judicial voyeurism" and just does not make sense.

There is a second type of test that can be used in a court, and I have called it personal rather than legal because all of us can apply it to ourselves, whether we are acting as doctors, family members, next of kin, or guardians. It is the test of substituted judgment, which says that we are going to do "x" not because we believe it is in the patient's best interests, because the doctors think it is in their best interests, or because the family thinks it is in its best interests, but rather because we think it is what that patient would do if the patient were capable of making a decision. This in many ways is almost a sillier test, even though I agree with it philosophically as an advocate of informed consent, as one who believes that people should be treated the way they want to be treated. However, in the substituted-judgment test, we are not dealing with competent people. Competent people are relatively easy—we do what they tell us to do, assuming that they understand the situation and know what is best for them. But with incompetent people, how do we ever know what they would have wanted to do?

Actually, we do not know (unless somehow they could tell us beforehand, as through a living will). When we talk about patients who never had a living will, such as infants, newborns, and people who have been mentally retarded all their lives—people who never have had an opportunity to make any major decisions about themselves or their lives—the answer is that we simply do not know what they would choose. We have no way of telling, and therefore we are not really substituting judgment in the sense of saying what they would do. We have gone back to saying what we think they should do, what I as a judge, what I as a doctor, or what I as a guardian believe this person should do. In effect, this process has not taken us anywhere, although in theory it is a very nice idea. I would imagine that the reason the substituted-judgment test is used is not because we believe it is realistic—clearly it is not—but because it makes us feel better. Ethical comfort is something we all seek in these decision-making processes. It is one of the main purposes of ethics committees, for example. When several people are involved, no one person actually makes the decision, and everybody goes home believing "we" did the right thing: "I didn't do it. Somebody else took responsibility for making that decision."

If we were to take substituted judgment seriously, for instance, we would need to go to court both when we were and when we were not going to treat patients. A hearing would have to be held every time a major decision was going to be made for every patient. No one has suggested this procedure, as Judge Liacos substantiated earlier. And since this suggestion has never been made, I would conclude that substituted judgment is something the court never took very seriously.

It seems to me that perhaps the *Saikewicz* court introduced substituted judgment because it thought that the decision made by the lower court was wrong. The judges might have been asking themselves, as Prof. Burt intimated, "How can we justify not treating this cancer patient solely because he is mentally retarded?" The answer is that such a decision cannot be justified on the basis of best interests. In the case of Mr. Saikewicz, for example, the court could have said he would be better off dead only if they added "because he is mentally retarded," and the court was not willing to do that. Therefore, the only way the law could ever publicly justify nontreatment for a mentally retarded person like Mr. Saikewicz would be to say that he is better off dead because if he could have made the decision himself, he would have declined treatment. This, of course, is complete fiction.

Without substituted judgment, however, we would be setting up two categories of patients, the first mentally retarded and the second not mentally retarded, and treating them differently, which is precisely what the *Saikewicz* court rightly said cannot be done. The judges used substituted judgment not because they felt that was the way all cases should be decided, but because this was the way that case had to be decided so as not to look as if they were treating mentally retarded people differently. My point is not that neither the best interests test nor the substituted-judgment test is serviceable, but only that both have major conceptual or practical problems. Judicial review, where used, may accordingly be more appropriately and honestly based on a simple determination that the contemplated action is "fair and reasonable" under the circumstances.

Let me conclude with a quotation from Harvard University's 1978 commencement speaker, Alexander Solzhenitsyn, who warned, in his much maligned address, that while a society without any objective legal scale is "terrible," "a society with no other scale but the legal one is not quite worthy of man either."

> A society that is based on the letter of the law and never reaches any higher is taking small advantage of the high level of human possibilities. The letter of the law is too cold and formal to have a beneficial influence on society. Whenever the tissue of life is woven of legalistic relations, there is an atmosphere of mediocrity paralyzing man's noblest impulses.

I submit that exactly this kind of paralysis has occurred in Massachusetts after *Saikewicz*. For example, I have heard of individuals who are brain dead being put on respirators and continually being resuscitated; terminally ill children with diseases like Tay-Sachs and Wernig-Hoffman's syndrome being heroically and painfully maintained; a dying woman being defibrillated 70 times in a 24-hour period; and relatives physically blocking and barring doors to prevent resuscitation teams from working over their loved ones. Such situations are outrageous. They are an overreaction to *Saikewicz* that exemplifies the worst in legalistic thinking.

It is my hope, and I think the hope of most of us here, particularly after hearing Judge Liacos, that we can go beyond this. I hope we can become more reasonable and realistic in our expectations about immunity. Professionals must act responsibly rather than authoritatively, and we must all work together to be realistic in our approaches to dying patients. Let us stop screaming and yelling at each other about why someone is wrong, or how we read the case, or why we do or do not have to go to court.

Another valuable thing to keep in mind is that different people have different interests, and we need to look at the perspectives of the various individuals concerned. In particular, we have to distinguish hospitals from doctors. Physicians, in many ways, have been treated unfairly, for they have been portrayed as desiring total immunity and being unwilling to do anything unless they have this guarantee. In fact, in looking at the cases that have gone to court, it is more often than not the hospital or hospital administrator who is insisting on total immunity; it is not the medical profession or the nursing profession that is pressing for these guarantees. Certainly, there are grounds for discussion, and I am optimistic that progress is being made and that the stage of acceptance is drawing nearer.

NOTES

1.   For a more detailed discussion of the *Quinlan* and *Saikewicz* cases and other matters raised in this chapter, see G. J. Annas, Reconciling *Quinlan* and *Saikewicz:* decision making for the terminally ill incompetent. *Am. J. Law Med.* 4:367–396, 1979.

2.   It is worth noting that in emergency situations, courts are very sympathetic to physicians and will, indeed, expect them to treat the patient first and ask questions later. Good-faith decisions as to what constitutes an emergency will be accepted by the courts as rightly a medical decision that should not be second-guessed under normal circumstances.

3.   R. Mnookin. Child-custody adjudication: judicial functions in the face of indeterminacy. *Law Cont. Prob.* 39:227, 1975.

The Michigan Medical Treatment Decision Act

Bruce L. Miller, Ph.D.

15

In the ordinary case of a physician treating a competent adult patient, the physician recommends treatment for the patient and the patient accepts it. The desire of patients to get well and their trust in physicians mean that patients seldom refuse recommended treatment. However, patients have the right to refuse treatment. This right is contained in the doctrine of informed consent, a legal doctrine based on every individual's right to self-determination. Obtaining the informed consent of a patient requires that the physician inform the patient of the proposed procedure, explain the risks and benefits of the procedure, as well as any alternatives, including not treating the patient, and then receive the patient's voluntary permission to do the procedure. This doctrine is well established in common law, although matters of detail remain uncertain, such as how much information must be given.

Medical decision making for competent adult patients is clear and well established; the roles of patient and physician are neatly set out. But if a patient is not competent, the legal waters become murky. This is true for patients who have never been competent, such as minors and adults who are severely mentally infirm, and for patients who were once competent but have lost that competence by reason of coma, unconsciousness, profound senility, or a devastating terminal illness.

One of the great moral concerns of the past few decades is the constellation of fears of medical treatment decisions, which has produced a great interest in "natural death" and "death with dignity." These slogans and the movements behind them point to the increasing power of medicine to maintain life—sometimes beyond the hope of recovery of any form of sapient status. In addition to the technological imperative, "if it can be done, it will be done," medicine has provoked such a strong response to its increased power for two other reasons. First, when patients are no longer competent and thereby not able to accept or refuse treatment, the decision-making procedures lose the clarity that the doctrine of informed consent provides. Who makes decisions when patients are no longer able to do so? Should decisions be controlled by patients' previous expressions of their wishes, where available; should the closest family member make the decision; or should it be the physician who decides? If the physician and the next of kin are each thought to have an equal voice, what happens if they disagree? The second reason is that in response to the uncertainty of decision-making authority, physicians are inclined to continue treatment. When no effective voice exists to say "no," their view that the dominant end of medicine is to preserve life will urge them to try every technique.

The two classes of patients mentioned above—the never competent and the once competent—present very different problems for medical decision making. Many proposals for decision procedures for the latter class of patients have been put forth. The Michigan Medical Treatment Decision Act is one such proposal. The process in which it evolved is as interesting as its content.

In 1976, Rep. David Hollister established the Task Force on Death and Dying, which is one of several such groups. Membership is open to any citizen who wishes to participate. Its function is to study the issues within its title and to recommend legislation or other government action as appropriate. Given the method of the group's composition, there was no specific and continuing membership. There was, however, a stable core of members. This included physicians, nurses, hospital administrators, lawyers, philosophers, interested citizens, senior citizens, and representatives of state agencies, the medical society, and the bar association. Every reasonable attempt was made to ensure that all individuals or groups who had an interest were able to know what was being considered by the task force and to participate if they desired. In addition to regularly scheduled meetings, some members of the task force made presentations to civic, religious, and professional groups.

The task force began with a detailed study of the California Natural Death Act, which had recently been enacted and was receiving attention throughout the country. The bill provides for a legally effective living will. A person may sign a directive instructing a physician not to continue treatment when that person's death is imminent, whether medical treatment is given or not. The task force wrestled with the details of the California bill for many meetings. Barry Keene, the assemblyman who sponsored the California bill, visited Michigan to discuss it. Eventually, problems with the bill led some members of the task force to reject the California approach in favor of a legislative approach suggested by Robert Veatch in *Death, Dying, and the Biological Revolution.* Rather than clarification via anticipatory decision making by the patient, Veatch argues for clarification via patient appointment of an agent to make medical decisions when the patient becomes unable to do so.

Argument on these two approaches was intense and protracted. To determine a course of action, two groups within the task force were assigned to draft a version for each approach; following this, the two drafts were considered by the task force and a vote taken to settle on one of them as the bill that would be further refined for legislative action. The agent approach suggested by Veatch was narrowly supported by the task force and was revised, refined, and rewritten many times before it was put on the docket of the Michigan Public Health Committee.

The process throughout was not political in the pejorative sense; that is, it was not a matter of competing interest groups using their political influence to push for a bill with minimal disadvantage to their authority. Rather, the process was political in the honorific sense, in that members of the public with an interest in medical decision making came together to forge a piece of legislation that responded to the issues and the concerns of the many subgroups of the public. It was marked throughout by mutual respect, and everyone involved was educated by those with a different approach or set of experiences.

The bill that emerged from this process has three major objectives, in response to three major concerns. The first objective is to enhance and extend an individual's right to accept or refuse treatment, to exercise the right to self-determination in the medical context. The task force agreed that the wishes of the patient should be dominant when treatment decisions have to be made. Incompetent patients should not become the mere object of the decision of others. Second, decision-making procedures should be clarified and uniform. Every hospital has some sort of procedure for indicating when a patient should not be resuscitated, referred to as no-code or do not resuscitate policies and procedures. One difficulty with them is that they vary tremendously from one hospital to another and, within a hospital, from one physician to another. Third, the question of liability for physicians, hospitals, and family members should be resolved. Great uncertainty exists in most states, including Michigan, on when a physician or hospital would be liable for not continuing treatment without express refusal by the patient. Furthermore, it is possible that a family member might be liable for a decision to discontinue treatment.

The objectives of the legislation are realized in the following major provisions, the first of which is quoted directly from the current bill:

1. "An adult person has the right to accept or refuse medical treatment in accordance with that person's wishes or desires. This right includes a refusal of medical treatment which would extend the person's life.

   "An adult person may appoint an agent who will act on behalf of the appointer if, due to a condition resulting from illness or injury and in the judgment of the attending physician, the appointer becomes incapable of making a decision in the exercise of the right to accept or refuse medical treatment."

2. A format for a document appointing an agent is provided in the bill; it includes the possibility of an alternate agent in the event that the first-mentioned person is unavailable.

3. There are provisions for a person to revoke an appointment and for an individual to refuse, at any time, to be the agent of another.

4. Agents, physicians, and other health care professionals are protected from liability for actions taken under the provisions

of the bill, providing they act in good faith and not in violation of civil and criminal law.

5. Physicians and other health care professionals are bound to the decisions of an agent by a provision that specifies that failure to comply with them imports the same legal liability that would obtain if the decision had been made by the appointing patient.

The above provisions respond to the major concerns that have been voiced about medical decision making for once-competent patients. Once they were accepted as the heart of the legislation, three problems with which the task force had to deal emerged.

First, the most common criticism of the bill, which was, however, not a denial of its basic idea, was what members of the task force came to call "the problem of the abusive agent." It was usually presented by descriptions of unlikely, but worrisome, scenarios. For example, suppose an individual is stricken with an illness or injury that, although it does not seriously threaten life or indicate a "vegetative" existence, renders that person incapable of making a medical decision; if the patient is given appropriate treatment, recovery at the least will be to a condition in which death is not imminent and the patient's mental and physical capacities permit a life of significant awareness and meaningful relationships. But now imagine that the agent appointed by the patient directs the physician to discontinue or not start treatment, without which the patient will die. The agent may be acting from a consciously held malicious motive or, what is more likely, from a belief that the patient would prefer not to be treated or that the patient would be better off not treated. Either reason could appear to the physician or others to have no or little basis and therefore to have emanated from unexamined feelings of the agent that are hostile, fearful, protective, escapist, or something else that would explain the agent's misunderstanding of the patient's condition and prospects.

In most cases like this, discussion among the physician, the agent, and other involved parties would resolve the situation. The "abusive agent" would be persuaded that discontinuing treatment is not in the interest of the patient. For those situations in which the agent is steadfast in the refusal of treatment, a physician or relative of the patient may request an expedited hearing before a circuit court to remove the agent temporarily or permanently. The plaintiff in such an action must show that the agent's decision is not "in accordance with the degree of care reasonably expected of a person who has a duty to act in good faith and with due regard for the interest and benefit of the appointing person."

The need to provide a court hearing for cases like that described is sometimes taken to show that legislation with regard to medical decisions cannot resolve the dilemmas associated with them and therefore is needless. But no legislation, on any topic, provides an easy way to reach a noncontroversial solution to every case imaginable. There will always be difficult, if not intractable, cases; the test of legislation is not whether it will make the worst possible cases simple, but whether it will contribute to a resolution of the problems in the more common and less difficult situations. There are easy cases that do not require legislation, and there are hard cases that legislation cannot make easy; between these extremes are the cases that require legislation and will be clarified by legislation.

The second problem concerns the status of living wills. The basic approach of the proposed legislation is that the appointment of an agent is a more effective way to extend an individual's right to accept or refuse treatment beyond the point when that individual is no longer competent. The California approach, which makes living wills legally effective, was rejected by our group because the generality and vagueness of such documents put the real decision-making authority in the hands of the person to whom the living will is addressed. Nonetheless, living wills are widely accepted; many people have made them out, and many more contemplate doing so. Thus, support existed for providing some recognition of living wills in the legislation. There is no problem with recognizing living wills provided that no legal penalty can be imposed for not following them, for to hold a person liable for not acting in accord with a document whose very nature makes it extremely difficult to determine when it has or has not been followed is an imposition of a legal burden without legal clarification.

To recognize living wills without at the same time creating ambiguous responsibilities, the Michigan bill says that it "shall not preclude an adult person from preparing written instructions for his or her medical treatment" and that living wills are "advisory and are evidence of the person's wishes and interests." It is further provided that an agent's decision shall prevail over written instructions and that if there is no agent, a physician is not liable for acting in accord with written instructions if doing so does not violate civil or criminal law.

The third problem involves emergency medical treatment. Initially, no provision was made for it because we thought that the existing common law exempting a physician from the requirement to obtain patient consent when the patient is incompetent and in need of emergency treatment would be transferable with regard to an agent. Enough concern arose over this, however, that an express provision was made. The authority of an agent is not required in "an emergency situation where medical care is needed to stabilize the patient's condition in response to an unanticipated, active illness or injury."

One major aspect of legislation of this sort does not appear in the current version of the Michigan bill. In Robert Veatch's draft, a provision states that if an individual has not appointed an agent, then the decision-making authority falls to a relative of the first degree of kinship, and if no such relative exists or is available, then to a relative of the second degree of kinship, and so on. Thus, there would be a designated decision maker for everyone. The Michigan bill is permissive. If an agent is not appointed and a person becomes incompetent, there is no clarification of the decision-making procedure and no enhancement of that person's right to accept or refuse medical treatment. The situation for such a patient would be no different from that without legislation. An early draft of the Michigan bill contained a section specifying a descending order of decision makers for every patient who becomes incompetent. The language was modeled on a provision of the Uniform Anatomical Gift Act, which stipulates a descending order of relatives with the authority to consent to anatomical gifts from a deceased person. This section was removed because of the argument of some members of the task force that since everyone would be covered with such a section in the bill, medical decision-making procedures were determined for all people whether they wanted it or not, and this was an untenable interference with their liberty.

Other members of the task force, while not persuaded by this argument, favored deletion, because doing so would make it easier to pass the bill. If it can be argued that a proposed piece of legislation will affect those who wish to take advantage of it and not affect those who see no advantage in it, it is politically easier to pass the bill. Still other members believed that the section did not constitute a real threat to liberty and that having a bill that would cover all cases was important enough to introduce it with that provision, but they were willing to delete if it became clear that doing so would significantly increase the chance that the bill would pass. This last group was not able to persuade the other two groups, and the permissive version of the bill was adopted by the task force.

The Medical Treatment Decision Act was introduced in the Public Health Committee of the Michigan House of Representatives late in the 1978 legislative session. Public hearings were held, but no action was taken by the committee. It was reintroduced in the 1979 session but not voted out, because of the absence of a member and a consequent tie vote. At this time, August 1979, Rep. Hollister hopes to have another vote in the Public Health Committee, with all members present, or to introduce the bill in another house committee or through the senate. Strong opposition to the bill is coming from antiabortion organizations, who regard it as not pro-life. The bill may not reach the floor of the house or the senate in this session, and if it does, it may not pass. But that will not be a complete loss; the attention focused on the bill has clearly enhanced the public's awareness and understanding of the dilemmas of medical decision making. That sort of result is a definite advance.

Legislative Inertia on Nontreatment Legislation

Sen. Louis P. Bertonazzi

16

Legislation for nontreatment decisions in Massachusetts is currently focusing on proposals for a so-called living will, which would enable patients, if incapacitated, to refuse heroic treatment at the time of imminent death and to do so beforehand in a document of approved legal form that provides immunity from liability for physicians who cooperate with the directives of such a document.

The present legislative session in Massachusetts is considering two bills on nontreatment, both of the living will genre. Even though a great deal of concern—indeed, a certain amount of turmoil—about nontreatment decision making exists in Massachusetts, these proposed laws have no serious chance of enactment. The fact is that, at this time, all real movement toward such legislation is at a virtual standstill.

Such a phenomenon regarding issues of public import is not in itself unusual. That such a phenomenon can exist, however, is generally not understood by outsiders to the political process, who often assume that because such matters are fueled by public concern and interest, they will proceed on their merits through rational advancement to a logical conclusion reflective of public consensus. Actually, legislators rarely have a clear and definitive assessment of public opinion regarding a matter such as nontreatment. Even public opinion polls and referendum questions, if they were to be exercised here, would depend heavily for their results on the manner and technique in which the question was posed.

Instead of public opinion, legislative decision making is generally more dependent on (and susceptible to) the lobbying efforts of well-organized interest groups, which are potent through the fruits of their organization: information, money, access to the public through media, and their resultant power to punish or reward legislators. In this respect, it is important to understand that the voting public in Massachusetts organizes to punish or reward legislators only every two years at the polls, while a well-organized interest group can exert its influence on even a daily basis. Therefore, the interest group is able to impose a much richer and more specific schedule of punishment or reinforcement than the general public, whose schedule is comparatively thin and, as a rule, not contingent on legislative behavior.

Clearly, the interest group, organized, financed, and motivated around specific issues, is a more powerful vehicle for influence than is an amorphous voting public. Skinner's comment relating to the group (society) and controlling agency (government) might well be extended to include the same relativity of organization between the legislature and interest group:

> The group exercises ethical control over each of its members through its power to reinforce or punish. The power is derived from sheer number and from the importance of other people in the life of each member. Usually, the group is not well organized, nor are its practices consistently sustained. Within the group, however, certain *controlling agencies* manipulate particular sets of variables. These agencies are often better organized than is the group as a whole, and they often operate with greater success.[1]

This is not to say, however, that legislators are incapable of sensing issues that generate concern and interest in the public at large. The question is the creation of interest in a specific ethical concern, which may be broached in a legislator's constituency by anyone with the motivation and means to do so: the legislator as an individual, the press, an already established institution, or an organized interest group. On occasion, all of them will compete in the creation of specific public opinion, and the voters will become the recipients of a plethora of information, opinions, appeals to authority, and the like.

More often than not, however, the public at large is bypassed and is left with its broad, unspecified concern about a particular issue. When this is the case, the interest groups, without bothering to create specific opinions in the general constituency, nonetheless behave as if they have created (or can create) such opinions. They proceed to influence legislative behavior on this basis, using their immediate day-to-day contingencies while being backed by the most potent contingency, that of creating a specific attitude in the constituency that will be translated into rewarding or punishing votes on election day.

For nontreatment—and the present issue in Massachusetts, living wills—the general public's concern and interest are yet unspecified. At the same time, though, activity to influence legislation has begun by interest groups. The result of this activity is the present standstill in nontreatment legislation in Massachusetts.

To understand why, we need to view the situation from two perspectives, the first historical (that is, the approach to the "right to die" and its context as they have developed in Massachusetts) and the second functional (that is, the specific organizations, structures, and processes extant formally and informally for enactment of law in the Massachusetts legislature).

Historically, nontreatment and right-to-die issues reached the point of serious discussion in the Massachusetts legislature during the 1978 session, at about the same time medical malpractice insurance become an issue. Other states were seeing drastic increases in malpractice premiums, and local physicians feared similar increases here unless prophylactic legislation was enacted. Physicians believed that attorneys' practices were at the root of the problem, while the legal profession believed that there was need for improvement in patient care by physicians. Both professional groups complained that insurance underwriters were less than candid in explaining the money and risk issues in the situation. In addition, hospital administrators registered their obvious concerns, also having a stake in the determination of liability.

Discussion of the malpractice situation naturally led to a

broader consideration of the issue of professional responsibility. Although the Massachusetts legislature by now had produced reasonable first-step legislation dealing with malpractice, which established some boundaries for the problem, issues about the dilemmas of dying had arisen during these discussions. No doubt, these issues were intensified and sharpened by the aftermath of the *Quinlan* case in New Jersey and the *Saikewicz* case in Massachusetts, both in 1976. The national press also became actively interested in the subject, for example, with *Newsweek* printing an extensive examination of death with dignity, relying heavily on interviews with hospice advocates and the work of psychiatrist Elisabeth Kübler-Ross. The public as a whole was well aware at this time of the issue as a matter of some concern, and this concern was fundamental to its crystalization into serious legislative discussion in 1978, triggered initially by the malpractice issue.

The malpractice issue is important here in another respect. When the dilemmas of dying situation reached serious discussion, significant interest groups—representing physicians, lawyers, and hospitals—were at work in the legislative field, called out initially by the malpractice matter. In Massachusetts, these groups are represented by the Massachusetts Medical Society, the Massachusetts Bar Association, and the Massachusetts Hospital Association.

None of these groups had a definitive and comprehensive legislative program for nontreatment decision making, although all of them registered a sense (reminiscent of the unfocused and broad public concern) that responsibility in the area needed procedural definition. This kind of definition, however, is never adequate to evoke and sustain serious legislative behavior. For issues such as nontreatment, the legislature is always passive and inactive without both a well-defined proposal and an organized effort to impose contingencies that reinforce or punish legislative behavior or the lack of it. The Massachusetts Medical Society and the Massachusetts Hospital Association did sponsor legislation around the issue of incompetence to refuse medical treatment but later withdrew support when a court decision was handed down in favor of their position.

In short, in 1978 there existed broad public concern about nontreatment decision making and an undefined but vocal sense by the interest groups representing physicians, lawyers, and hospitals that responsibility in nontreatment decisions required procedural definition, but none of these groups was committed to a definitive legislative program to the extent of exercising their considerable influence on the legislature. The malpractice issue had brought the organized groups to the legislature, but there seemed to be a reluctance to deal beyond this issue with the nontreatment corollary in a more than general way of discussion and tentative legislative initiatives.

On June 20, 1977, the U.S. Supreme Court handed down a decision that was to result in the heightened presence of another major interest group in the Massachusetts legislative arena. This was the decision in *Maher* v. *Rowe*, which established that the equal protection clause of the U.S. Constitution did not require states to expend monies through welfare payments for abortions and that such expenditures were the prerogative of the states through democratic process, which meant decision making in the legislatures. In Massachusetts a prolonged and hard-fought legislative battle followed, culminating in victory for the abortion opponents with passage of the Doyle-Flynn amendment on July 8, 1978, which prohibited use of welfare funds and state employee health plans for abortions.

The adoption of Doyle-Flynn was tremendously significant. Those familiar with Massachusetts politics know that, as a result of the abortion issue, the major right-to-life group here—Massachusetts Citizens for Life, Inc.—has had the strongest impact on legislation and legislators of any single interest group established in recent years. This organization, which began as an ad hoc group to oppose abortion referendum questions in 1972, was incorporated in 1973 and to date has established 89 chapters across the state, according to its present president. The group sends information to a mailing list of 60,000 members and interested persons. The Massachusetts Medical Society, on the other hand, has a membership of 9,813, organized into 21 district societies, while the Massachusetts Bar Association has 10,910 members, and the Massachusetts Hospital Association represents 180 institutions.

At present, these last three groups have not taken positions as organizers on nontreatment decision making beyond the present practices arising out of common law, although their concern for the establishment of some procedural methodology is evident in discussions by their legislative representatives. But the Massachusetts Citizens for Life presents a very definite position on nontreatment: strenuous opposition to living wills or any legislation that "would give the members of the medical profession legal immunity for any action taken after the patient was declared terminal."[2] This organization further relates living will legislation to the euthanasia issue, a relationship cited by its former president, Katherine P. Healey, as already having been made by the Concern for Dying organization in an October 3, 1978, letter from the latter group's executive director: "It is this close relationship which has prompted many to see the living will as the first step towards the ultimate legislation of euthanasia, which is currently classified as homicide."[3]

The interests of the medical, hospital, and legal professions in the issue, objectively examining their efforts to date in the legislature, are broad, undefined, and, in a sense, peripheral. On the contrary, the interest of Massachusetts Citizens for Life is direct, well defined, and unequivocal. Why this is so suggests some important lines of scholarly investigation concerning motivation, decision making, leadership makeup, and membership of organized groups. What is clear now, however, is that the Massachusetts Citizens for Life, richly reinforced and highly motivated from its stunning success in opposition to abortion, has clear and present ascendancy of the nontreatment and living will issues among interest groups at work in the Massachusetts legislature.

Given the structure of the legislature, formal and informal, the result is the current legislative standstill on nontreatment and living will issues, since it is interest groups, armed with research, well-defined proposals, day-to-day presence in legislators' offices and committee hearings, and imposing conditions specifically contingent on legislative behavior, that produce action (or inaction). For example, a bill in the present legislative session, initiated by a private citizen and calling for state income tax deductions for blood donors, died in committee, mostly owing to the opposing efforts of the American Red Cross, the acknowledged "owner" of matters relating to blood donation. On the other hand, the American Red Cross was unable to prevent the passage of legislation allowing certain commercial enterprises to establish services for blood collection; the lobbying efforts of the enterprises were more effective. The point here is that the legislative structure is not geared to a rational exposition of the issue at hand. Instead, it yields to the push and pull of interest groups operating in a legislature that, regarding issues, is essentially *tabula rasa*. This is true with only minor exceptions and unless legislators' constituencies have made their positions highly specific and are overwhelmingly polarized.

It is clear, therefore, that the future of nontreatment and living will legislation in Massachusetts is negative if the present situation continues. What would be required to change this situation is the emergence of new interest groups in favor of the legislation or its adoption by one or more already established groups. These groups would then have to pursue one or both of the following courses: (1) a massive, day-to-day effort in the legislature, using all the tools that such groups have at their disposal, and (2) a massive effort to polarize legislators' constituencies into specific behaviors indicative of approval. The ethical rightness or wrongness of the matter is insufficient to produce action, and the advantage belongs to those who desire the present situation.

NOTES

1.   B. F. Skinner. *Science and human behavior.* New York: The Free Press, 1978, p. 333.

2.   Letter from Massachusetts Citizens for Life, Inc., to members, Massachusetts House of Representatives, April 30, 1979.

3.   Letter from Katherine P. Healey, then president, Massachusetts Citizens for Life, Inc., to members, Joint Committee on the Judiciary, Massachusetts General Court, October 3, 1978.

BIBLIOGRAPHY

Ferster, C. B.; Culbertson, S.; and Perrott Boren, M. C. *Behavior principles,* 2nd ed. Englewood Cliffs, N.J.: Prentice-Hall, 1975.

Horan, D. J. Euthanasia and brain death: ethical and legal considerations. In *Studies in law and medicine,* vol. 1. Chicago: Americans United for Life, Inc., 1977.

Horan, D. J., and Marzen, T. J. Death with dignity and the "living will." In *Studies of law and medicine,* vol. 4. Chicago: Americans United for Life, Inc., 1978.

Living with dying. *Newsweek.* May 1, 1978.

Roundtable Discussion

John A. Robertson, J.D., Moderator

17

Mr. Neil L. Chayet (Attorney, Warner & Stackpole, Boston):
We are at the point now where we have to admit that the situation
is horrendous. In fact, it is deteriorating, and we are being left with
further uncertainties. I am sure that Judge Liacos really believes that
he did the right thing, and perhaps it is the only thing that he could
have done in the name of protecting the public interest. But what is
the public interest? It is one more example of a very difficult
concept to define.

Many court decisions are being based on the best interests of
a person; that, too, is not clear-cut. I found it shocking when I had
to go to court on behalf of a family of an infant with a disorder in
which the brain was unimpaired but every muscle of the newborn
baby was slowly being destroyed by disease. I intended to frame my
pleadings *in re*, but the judge told me that I must make the parents
the plaintiff and the baby the defendant. When I argued that the
parents did not want to sue their own baby, the judge replied that a
guardian ad litem was necessary, and furthermore, I would have to
serve papers on the baby. I would have to go to the hospital and
place the papers right on the baby or on the incubator. In this
particular case, as I was on my way to the hospital, the baby died. I

went anyway, and I would urge every judge and lawyer involved in this area to do the same. You have to go only once, but you should see what is being done in the hospitals. You need to understand that this is not strictly an academic legalistic exercise; you need to get a taste of the difficulty of the decisions that are being made.

Now, in light of *Saikewicz*, what is the answer? The only sure thing is that we cannot go home again. I personally would have preferred that such decisions remained with physicians, although I would like to see physicians better trained in communications skills. Many other solutions have also been proposed, but they seem to raise further questions. After *Saikewicz*, doctors believed they could get their former decision-making powers back merely by telling the legislature that they wanted them back. However, as Sen. Bertonazzi pointed out, that is not going to happen, at least in Massachusetts. I found his remarks very discouraging. Those who seek a legislative solution have to start talking to their "opponents"; they cannot be ignored.

Another proposed solution is to set up ethics or prognosis committees, as in the *Quinlan* case. Hospital associations like this idea. It came as no surprise to me, however, that once the committee was formed after *Quinlan*, it could not reach a decision. The chances of a committee consisting of a physician, a lawyer, a hospital administrator, and someone from the clergy ever reaching a decision are almost minimal.

The agent concept, as explained by Prof. Miller, is an interesting one. My quick reaction, however, is that it merely moves the whole problem to another level. How can we choose agents when discord and conflict in the American family are so rampant? General practice lawyers now spend half their time in domestic relations. Should a spouse be chosen as an agent today when that spouse may be gone tomorrow?

Much of what Prof. Gadow said was good, except for one problem. The moment we say "patient advocate," we have begun to destroy what we are seeking to create. I know this is heresy for a lawyer to say, but I think the advocacy system, particularly in these areas, has run its course. In fact, as Prof. Burt said, it seems to bring about a paradoxical inverse result to what we seek.

Now that I have shot holes in everyone else's propositions, let me add that I fully agree that physicians do need help. I am uncomfortable with the suggestion that they should continue to take risks. I don't like the tone of today's lawsuits, and I am afraid that risk taking could very well be used against physicians. We have to provide some measure of protection for those whom we are asking to take these very difficult steps and make these very difficult decisions.

I would like to see a way in which we can have minimum intrusion but legal sufficiency so that we can move toward a reasonable solution. I submit one possibility, which I call a patient representative system. This system would be quite simple. The representative would work in and be paid by the hospital. While some may argue that this constitutes a conflict of interest, I believe that almost no one is totally free of conflict of interest. This person would also report regularly to the probate court. Now that the courts are involved in this area, they will not leave it, so the solution is to keep them involved but in a minimal way. The representative would be a skilled communicator, perhaps a nurse or a specially trained individual, who will help the exchange of information between the patient and the professionals. The real problem is not competence but rather determining what the information is and ensuring that patients get all the information they need. Another task of the representative, which is one of the things judges are most concerned about, would be to watch for signs of someone giving consent to get rid of a patient.

Assuming we have such an individual, that person would have one thing that nobody now has, and that is the legal authority to do something. Right now, many physicians are doing things that would have to be viewed as illegal. At the moment, it is believed that if the next of kin says that nontreatment is O.K., then it is O.K. That is simply not lawful at this time; all that really means is that there is less likelihood of the physician being sued. In one state, Louisiana, the next of kin has this authority, but in no others that I know of can the next of kin sign nontreatment papers without a legal appointment. In addition, if a physician is dealing with someone who is seriously impaired, the fact that the person has not been deemed incompetent does not necessarily mean that the patient is competent to give informed consent, so physicians are still left in the dark.

The patient representative would have the authority to

certify that the appropriate information was duly exchanged insofar as possible, and once the representative certified something, it would be functional and legally binding. Also certified would be the statement that, to the best of the representative's knowledge, there is nothing that looks strange about the case, or there is no reason for further inquiry. Obviously, if the representative believed that a problem existed, the court would be called in, and a hearing would be held immediately. But almost all of these difficult cases would be able to go forward.

In essence, the system that I envisage—a patient representative or patient surrogate system—would facilitate the exchange of information, which is often not done very well right now, and then give some measure of protection. It maintains the dignity of the human beings involved; it avoids the substituting of judgment, which is only another form of paternalism; and it enables those closest to the patient, without specifically being named agents, to work with the representative or facilitator to bring about an appropriate, fair, and equitable result.

Prof. Robertson: I noted what sounded like a contradiction in Prof. Burt's remarks. On the one hand, he seemed to suggest that there is something seriously wrong with denying medical care to a retarded person when any normal individual would have received that care. At the same time, he seems to castigate, or at least be critical of, the courts for being involved in this area. Yet, if the doctors and the superintendent of Belchertown had not been legally required to go to court, how would the interests of retarded patients have been protected?

It seems to me that going to court was precisely what was needed to determine and protect the interests of retarded individuals, and Prof. Burt placed a great deal of emphasis on the necessity of such protection. It may turn out, as he suggested, that the *Saikewicz* court erred in withholding care, but the idea of going to court was not at all inappropriate.

What we really have to be clear about is what role the courts should take. We need to separate the role of courts in setting down general rules and principles to guide physicians and other professionals with regard to retarded patients from the perhaps less necessary role of judges actually being involved in individual applications of the broad rules and principles. My sense is that Prof.

Burt would disagree with the idea of the courts actually applying the substantive rules in each case. I think I would too for the most part, but I believe that the courts should play a significant part in defining and laying down the broad substantive rules that are necessary to confine the exercise of professional judgment, particularly with regard to incompetent patients.

Prof. Burt: I quite agree with you; I was not arguing that the courts should not be involved. Indeed, it is critical that they take a very active role in protecting the interests of those groups who have been traditionally ignored, and those groups include not only the mentally retarded but perhaps patients as a whole as well. In promulgating informed consent, the courts have performed a very important function. Where I would call a halt to their involvement, as you indicated, is in a case-by-case application of those principles before anybody acts on them.

The real problem with the *Saikewicz* case was that there was no correct answer; either decision would have been wrong. That is the nature of moral dilemmas, and *Saikewicz* was the epitome of such a dilemma. In any legal or community decision, we must take care not to falsify what are true dilemmas. The difficulty in *Saikewicz* was that somebody had to decide, but when we turn that into a public decision, and when the decision says that it is proper not to treat this mentally retarded person in this circumstance, I disagree. I think it is a dangerous concept. Whichever way the decision went, it would be wrong. A court, however, cannot say that it cannot operate that way, and indeed it is hard for anyone to operate that way. In that kind of situation, what I would like to do is preserve an awareness of the dilemmatic qualities of true dilemmas.

Having said that, let me recognize another problem, and that is the problem of too much uncertainty, which is a point that Mr. Chayet also addressed. Moral dilemmas contain so much uncertainty that decisional capacities are themselves crippled. It seems to me that the kinds of decision-making mechanisms we should look for are those that do not leave us completely at sea. Mr. Chayet's idea of a patient representative is interesting, but I would hope that such a scheme would provide for quick access to the courts if anybody was troubled about a particular decision. Let's say this patient representative system gets started and then somebody sues; in this particular case, the court says that things look pretty reasonable. Then the next case comes along, and the patient representative has maybe 95 percent certainty that everything is O.K., but there is still the 5 percent that makes everybody worry. That is the amount of uncertainty that I want, 5 percent, not 95 percent. Unfortunately, Massachusetts right now is living with 95 percent uncertainty; that cannot remain, I agree. The danger is in seeking 100 percent certainty about things that just cannot be certain.

Mr. Ronald Schram (Attorney, Ropes and Gray, Boston): While it is possible to provide a means for getting before a court very promptly, these issues are so complex that their resolution may take a great deal of time. The *Saikewicz* case itself took 18 days before the lower court reached a decision; *McNulty* took 35 days; and the *Dinnerstein* case, which involved a do not resuscitate order—probably the situation with the most acute need for speed—took two and a half months from the date of filing to an initial decision. It is one thing to have prompt access to a court, and quite another to have a prompt decision by a court.

Prof. Robertson: Of course, part of the problem may be that the rules have not yet been laid down; we are still in the process of developing them. Perhaps the lengthy court process will be cut down once clearer rules and procedures are enunciated.

Dr. Mitchell T. Rabkin (General Director, Beth Israel Hospital, Boston): I am not sure that there was no right answer in *Saikewicz*. In fact, I wonder whether we have not altered the entire nature of the question that was being asked. I think it would have been, as Prof. Burt said, an impossible dilemma if Mr. Saikewicz had passively received the medical treatment, being as retarded as he was. The distinction is that there may have been only a medical decision and virtually no moral decision at all; in other words, the treatment was so incomprehensible to the patient and would have met with such resistance that it was deemed judicious from a clinical point of view not to do it. It would be as if somehow you were incarcerated against your will for reasons beyond your ken for, let's say, the prevention or treatment of some disability of which you were unaware. A physician, who might anticipate a horrible or deleterious event for you in the future, might at the same time recognize that to do all these things against your will, beyond your ken, for a consequence that you cannot even visualize and that will only cause you a tremendous amount of anguish over the period of treatment, would be an abuse of you as an individual. This might then cause the physician to say, clinically, "We are always taking risks and weighing one thing against the next. I deem this treatment to be inappropriate." I wonder whether, in fact, the medical profession in this instance was asking the court not what we have all been assuming all along—that is, for a rule on who makes the judgment in the case of an incompetent patient—but rather, for a clinical judgment.

We have now had two cases in which the individuality of the situation was not initially appreciated, and then things took off. That was certainly true in *Quinlan*. I submit that *Saikewicz* may not have been that kind of a moral dilemma. That does not, of course, ignore the existence of moral dilemmas. I merely want to point out the way we tend to proceed in a very specific case, as every one of these cases clearly must be.

Prof. Burt: I share your premise that what we seek are carefully individualized decisions. If Mr. Saikewicz had been subjected to the treatment, it was alleged that he would have resisted with all his might; he would have pulled the tubes out and would have thrashed about, and so on. There may have been other facts that were not introduced, but from my reading of the transcript, it seems clear that the degree of his resistance was excessively speculative and not adequately tested. The reason that I say excessive speculation is that the physician who testified about the impossibility of treatment saw Mr. Saikewicz at a tertiary treatment hospital and not in his home setting, the institution where he had lived nearly all his life. Of course he thrashed about and was impossible to deal with; he was a very scared and profoundly retarded man who was out of his accustomed environment.

Did the people who knew him on a day-to-day basis, those who cared for him daily and who were familiar to him, test out the treatment process in his own setting, or at least give it a try? My reading of the record shows that it was not tried. What about sedation? It was discussed in the abstract but was rejected on the grounds that sedation would introduce other adverse physical consequences, such as respiratory infection. How about trying just a little sedation? Granted, it would have been hard work and quite time-consuming, and Mr. Saikewicz was not a very rewarding patient. The question really was, "Why are we doing this? What is the benefit to be gained from all this extra effort?" Rather than testing to find out whether he would be passive or a wildly resistant beast, the issue was taken elsewhere to be resolved in the abstract. In other words, there was a premature freezing of what was at stake in order to have a judge decide what was right and what was wrong.

If the court had said, as well it might have, "We're not going to tell you, and you may indeed run a risk of subsequent liability," I could envision the following type of discussion. The physicians would go to their lawyers and say, "We do not want to treat Mr. Saikewicz, because he is going to resist." The lawyers, if they are worth anything, would reply, "I am imagining you on the stand, being prosecuted for homicide. The first question the prosecutor is going to ask is whether treatment was tried. If you say, 'No, it was not,' the prosecutor will then ask, 'How did you know Mr. Saikewicz would resist?'" In other words, the lawyers would advise the physicians to give treatment a try, to try to work further. The thing that is going to individualize this or any other case is the extra measure of effort. I do not think that anyone really knows the true individual characteristics of this particular decision. The physicians themselves got in the way of learning its true individual characteristics by simply going to court, and this was compounded by the court's willingness to take the case.

Dr. Frank Coco (Hematologist, Framingham Hospital, Framingham, Mass.): Although I do not purport to speak for any organization, I do work with the leukemia societies. It struck me in reading about the *Saikewicz* decision that there was a remarkable dearth of medical information about acute leukemia. While there is some dispute regarding the proper treatment, several points are generally agreed on. One is that adults, especially above the age of 60, although there is no specific age cutoff, do not respond to treatment for acute leukemia anywhere nearly so well as do children. The likelihood of success, therefore, is relatively remote if childhood leukemia is used as a comparative measure. A second point of agreement is that it is not possible to try a modest course of therapy, such as was possible in trying a couple of hours without a respirator in the *Quinlan* case, because you cannot give a touch of chemotherapy. This particular type of leukemia requires a very aggressive combination of drugs, and anything less than that is likely to be ineffective. It would thus not be reasonable to assume that a minimal wait-and-see type of action would really do anything, unless you are suggesting a sham course of therapy in which an intravenous is started just to see what the patient's responsiveness is, and I do not think that is what Prof. Burt was implying.

I also want to go back to Prof. Burt's earlier remarks. When we make assumptions about what an incompetent person wants, we consciously and sometimes subconsciously insert our own particular value judgments. We all tend to impose them, and I think Prof. Burt imposed one earlier when he said that competent patients would definitely and naturally want treatment for leukemia or any other cancer. This is not always so. Given the options and depending on how the data are presented, people may well choose not to take treatment, especially in view of the relatively poor response of adults; and the older the patient is, the more likely will be the need for supportive therapy, such as a respirator. I would submit that the basic assumption on Prof. Burt's part, which is shared by many people, is that if someone refuses treatment for something, that person must be crazy and therefore incompetent.

Prof. Burt: What I said was that, in court, everyone testified that almost all mentally normal people would accept chemotherapy; I did not say that was my own judgment. The judge decided the case on the assumption that mentally normal people would opt for treatment. Now, of course, that assumption can be debated, but what struck me as pernicious was the judge's willingness to assume that as a fact and nonetheless to decide contrary to that fact for this particular person.

Dr. Arnold Relman (Editor, *New England Journal of Medicine,* Boston): There seems to be a consensus that we are in a diffi-cult situation now. We cannot go back. We recognize that we cannot reverse time's arrow, but how are we going to get out of this situation? Prof. Burt seemed to suggest that we got into this position because of the doctors' failure of nerve, failure to accept the responsibility and liability inherent in the practice of medicine and in the decisions they must make. If that is true, is the way out simply to regain our nerve and start making the decisions again, while being prepared to accept the consequences? Shall we just let the chips fall where they may and not be intimidated by *Saikewicz* or other court decisions—in other words, more or less throw ourselves on the mercy of society's common sense and sense of fair play?

My own view is that Prof. Burt is only half right. We got into this pickle not just because of physicians' excessive concern for immunity, but because of a very important change in society's view of medicine and physicians. We have emerged from an era in which physicians and other professionals were deified, a time before consumerism and suggestions that physicians had limited knowledge or authority. Now we are in an era in which the doctors' authority and professionalism are being challenged (partly for good reason, in my opinion), a time when many very intelligent and very sophisticated people are attempting to distinguish between technical, medical decisions that doctors ought to make and moral, ethical decisions that doctors should not make. However, this distinction, which is exceedingly difficult to make, blurs when you examine it, particularly if you examine it with knowledge of what the practice of medicine really is. Perhaps it is philosophically defensible by someone who has never practiced medicine, but if you really know what doctors have to do, it is a distinction that you cannot maintain.

My point is that, in addition to the physicians' failure of nerve and their insistence on immunity, this troublesome situation has been caused by the increasing credence that many influential people in society are giving to the idea that doctors are technicians. They may be very expensive and very highly trained, but, as it does with airline pilots, the public will put its lives in their hands and pay them a lot of money because they know all about flying planes. In the same way, many people are leaving the technical details to physicians while maintaining that other important things related to medicine are none of the physicians' business. It seems to me that pressing this distinction too far is one of the causes of our current situation. Another, of course, is the general revolt against all authority. Physicians, having been among the most authoritative figures in our society, are now regarded with great suspicion and hostility.

My concern today, however, is how we get out of this pickle.

Is it possible, for example, that some overarching Supreme Court decision can be made that will resolve the issues, or are we going to have to see each of the 50 states, one at a time, painfully wrestle with this problem? When I was practicing in Philadelphia, for example, I had patients on both sides of the Delaware River. I had to treat my patients in Philadelphia differently from those in Camden, New Jersey, because I had to contend with different state laws. That is a horrible prospect. I would be delighted if all the states would develop something like the Michigan bill. While that bill clearly does not solve many of the problems, it solves some of them very well. It is an eminently sensible bill, in that it does not come down on one side or the other of the loaded issue of the right to die or the right to life. It concerns nothing but patients' rights, which is where the law ought to be.

Mr. Chayet: Although one might think that going to the Supreme Court would be a more rational approach, I would submit, after looking at recent Supreme Court decisions, that such a route would only make the situation worse. Legislatively, we already have problems here in Massachusetts, as described earlier. The Michigan law may be an approach to follow, but we should look at some of the other Michigan laws before we emulate it. Legislation is a mixed process, of course, but without question, a legislative approach is better than going through the courts.

If we are stymied in the courts and if we are stymied in the legislature, then what? Giving you a battlefied opinion, I would not recommend the route of civil disobedience in Massachusetts. In areas that are at all close to the issues that Sen. Bertonazzi talked about, there is a need to be very wary. Then comes the real question — what should physicians do when they believe that the route the law requires is not in the best interests of their patients or their profession? To act contrary to that route requires an act of courage. Physicians may get away with it, but as Dr. Relman pointed out, physicians are among the most unpopular people nowadays in the eyes of the courts, the legislature, and the press. Unfortunately, I think, physicians are a major target of antiprofessionalism.

I think that acting contrary to the law is very risky, and I would prefer that we come up with an alternative. We have to

mount a very significant legislative lobbying effort in Massachusetts. We should start negotiating with people we do not
ordinarily talk to, people who have a lot of power with the
legislature. Once we sit down with people, even those who have
different philosophies, we may find common pathways to achieve a
solution with which everybody can live. Remember, legislators are
patients, and judges are patients; the time has come to remind them
of that.

Prof. Annas: I would like to mention a couple of things that are not
helpful. One is to assume a hysterical attitude, believing that
everything is going to hell and everybody hates doctors, that we
have to get out the machine guns and do something horrible
because everybody is down on doctors. In truth, every public
opinion poll in the last two decades, including the most recent one,
shows that physicians are the most respected of all professionals.
The percentage is dropping, but most people have a great deal of
respect for physicians in general, and especially for their personal
physicians.

I also believe that it is not helpful to say that only doctors can
understand what doctors do. As Dr. Relman and others have put it,
"We know what doctors have to do, and no one else knows. There
is no way we can explain this. There is no way anyone else can ever
understand what it is to be a doctor." On some level, obviously, that
is true, just as no one can wholly understand what it is to be a bird
or any other type of creature unless one is that creature. But I do not
think it is helpful to keep saying that over and over again. In most
states, the medical licensing board is run by physicians. Clearly,
most legislatures believe that physicians primarily should say what
physicians do, but not exclusively. We are not going to turn back
the clock to a time of complete physician autonomy, because that
time may never have existed, and it certainly does not exist
anymore.

I do not think that the trust people have in doctors has
changed. What has changed is that people often no longer have
their own doctors. For example, in Dr. Todres's neonatal intensive
care unit, the infants are not his patients; they are all referred to him
from the community. The parents may know their personal
pediatricians, but they have probably never met Dr. Todres, so why
should they trust him? It is not that they do not trust doctors;

rather, it is that they do not know them. It takes time to develop trust.

Finally, I do not think that there is a magic bullet, and we should not look for one. It is silly for doctors to ask lawyers, judges, or legislators for simple or clear-cut answers, saying, "If we can get out of this in a clear way, then we don't have to worry about it anymore." It is like patients asking doctors to keep them alive forever, to cure the cancer, to do something to make it all go away. The answer is sometimes yes, sometimes no, and sometimes maybe.

We do have a solution for competent patients, and a very important one. Two state supreme courts have said that competent patients have the legal right to make their own decisions. Doctors can and should and, I would argue, are legally obligated to follow that law. If we had a living will bill, which I believe we should have, almost everyone would have the opportunity to take part in decisions. That would leave us with incompetent persons, some with and some without families, which are very difficult situations. I do not have the magic answer, nor does anyone. To lump all situations together and treat them all the same is not the way. With wards of the state and people without families, we know the answer; they need legal guardians, and they may or may not need court proceedings. The harder cases are the incompetent patients with families, and I think that Mr. Chayet is right—we need to experiment with different models. I do not believe that we are ready to write legislation dictating how it should always be done, nor is society ready to say how these decisions should be made. It is too soon. Actually, we do not really know what the lower court said in *Saikewicz*. Probably not even three or four people in this whole room have read the entire transcript. We must first do our homework and see what the law currently is before we decide how to change it.

Prof. Miller: Let me try to tie together what Prof. Burt was saying about the nature of moral dilemmas. I would prefer saying that there is no right answer, rather than that both answers are wrong. Whenever we put these decisions into a court context or any other context that presumes there is a right answer or a best answer by some measurable degree, we are making a mistake. Perhaps the most important thing is to know who made the decision, rather than which of the two decisions, both of which look equally unpalatable, has been made. This is what we are trying to get at in the Michigan bill. If it is a relatively straightforward situation, in which the physician recommends stopping the respirator or not resuscitating a comatose or nearly comatose, irreversibly ill person, and everyone agrees, then there will be no problem. Substantive standards can be made for cases like that. It is the less clear-cut cases that get very messy, for which all we can try to do is see that the correct procedures are followed, that the proper persons participate, and that the person with the final responsibility is the right person. Ideally, of course, the right person is the patient, the one with the most at stake. But since we can't ask the patient in the kind of cases we are talking about, we need to know who is next best, and that would be someone the patient trusts and would choose.

We cannot establish substantive standards for these difficult cases by court decisions, legislation, or living wills; the best we can do is get the right person to make the decision. That is the general idea of what we are trying to do in Michigan. If we can get people to understand that, by passage of legislation or otherwise, maybe some of these difficulties can be resolved.

Prof. Gadow: It would seem as if the evolution of the problem has been sketched out. The erosion of the authoritarian model of medicine is partly responsible. Even physicians have grown weary of the deity myth and are eager to relinquish it. On the other hand, physicians, quite rightly, are unwilling to accept the purely technical role, which I referred to as the consumerism model, in which they are strictly technical advisers and are required to delegate all value and ethical questions to courts, ethics committees, or perhaps patient representatives.

Between these two extremes, with which neither medicine nor patients are happy, lies a third alternative. To me, the answer is fairly obvious. We need a kind of fundamental philosophical change in medicine so that practitioners would become committed to practice what we might call collaborative medicine. I do not mean collaboration among greater numbers of specialists and subspecialists, but collaboration between medicine and the persons directly involved, primarily patients, but also families when available.

Unless this kind of basic philosophical commitment is articulated as the explicit ideal of medicine — and it is somewhat different from the traditional or historical ideals of medicine—the situation as it is now is simply going to continue. Medicine will be practiced authoritatively, on the one hand, and consumeristically or technically, on the other.

Sen. Bertonazzi: The kinds of decisions we are talking about are not new; they have been made for many, many years. But no one really discussed them before, and no one really cared a whole lot. I don't know whether the general public even wondered how decisions on death and dying were made. For the most part, they were simply made, and no one called for any kind of legislation. It was not until physicians felt that the public was watching them, which was not necessarily true but was perceived to be true, perhaps as a result of litigation, that a need was felt for some kind of legislation that would explain the directions physicians could take in these cases for their own protection.

There was a time when the public shared this view and did indeed demand that we move toward some kind of resolution. But then the public seemed to see the terrible complexity of the issues and to be scared off by it; as a result, there is far less pressure now for legislation, because of conflicts, than there was perhaps four or five years ago.

If legislation is the answer, the only method is to try to deal with one very small portion of it, rather than to develop legislation to address the issue in its entirety. I do not think that any of us is clear in the direction that such legislation should take. Rather, if legislation is felt to be needed, we should take an area in which agreement can be reached, not just between groups such as those here today, but among all groups that have an interest in the problem, regardless of the source of the interest. We would benefit more from limited legislation as a first step, so that we can learn from what we do, than from an attempt to come up with something we do not know enough about.

Dr. Rowell: I take issue with any implication that physicians are crazed killers trying to do away with patients; that is simply not true. What has brought us to this point is that we are getting into more moral dilemmas and thinking about them much more than in the past. I agree with Prof. Annas that judicial paternalism is no substitute for medical paternalism, but medicine is not so paternal as it used to be. It is more participatory. For example, look at the changes in obstetrics. The process used to be that a woman came into the hospital, was given extraordinary amounts of pain-killing drugs, had a baby, and that was that; it was a technical process. Now, it is a participatory process, with the father and the mother and even the other children involved.

I don't think the situation in Massachusetts is deteriorating; recent court decisions have brought us a different outlook. I am a little concerned about codification or going to the legislature to write out rules that tell us how to act in caring for the dying or terminally ill patient. It is almost impossible to write rules for every kind of situation. We have been dependent on common law because it is a reflection of our times. Oliver Wendell Holmes supported the view that jurisprudence, as it sweeps across our times, will change because we have changes in medically accepted practices. The practices now are different from 20 years ago.

Look at the example that Prof. Burt spoke about, Karen Quinlan and the problem of whether or not to take her off the respirator. The question was whether she satisfied all the criteria of brain death and she did not. If they had removed the respirator at a critical point in her illness, she would have died, but by weaning her from it slowly and gradually and finally removing it after all the litigation, she did survive without it. However, this has not changed the basic problem at all. Now we are left with a patient who is getting comfort and care, but her illness will be long and delayed. The particular situation has still not been addressed.

In Massachusetts, another important decision was the *Golston* case, which said that if a patient was dead by accepted medical criteria and standards, there was no question about shutting off the respirator. This was a court decision, and it works perfectly well. Another case, *Hall* v. *Myers*, involving an inmate, is probably going to be just as important as *Saikewicz* as far as its impact on our thinking and moral concerns about the rights of patients in giving or withholding treatment.

Dr. Prout: I have become increasingly upset as the morning has worn on, listening to proposed alternative solutions and trying to figure out what would happen to my terminal patients if each one of these was in effect. As I view these alternatives from my patients' perspectives, I find it unsettling, although maybe I am being "maternalistic." In our attempt to adjudicate or legislate or proscribe what are basically philosophical or metaphysical questions about the quality and value of life, I am perturbed that such decisions are going to be made by those of us who are healthy and who are basically winners in life. We must do a lot more homework concerning the people we are supposedly protecting before we can ever pretend to understand the range that we will have to encompass with our laws.

If I have learned anything from my years as an oncologist and from my numerous patients, it is how little I know philosophically about how much love and joy one can have even with a tenuous grip on life and lack of cerebration. As part of my responsibility, I personally accept the need for bringing these decisions out of the closet, and I would hope that others will accept the responsibility to come into my closet and see what we are dealing with. We are talking very intellectually about a lot of possibilities for which we really have not done the groundwork.

I am bothered that assumptions were made in *Saikewicz* regarding the patient's quality of life, with very little attempt made to improve that quality. In fact, I am anxious right now to go back to my patients and continue trying to improve their quality of life rather than debate it. This debate has not furthered my understanding of the quality of life. Much more can be done to improve this quality, and that will change what we might legislate or debate. The quality of life in *Saikewicz* was not considered very imaginatively; recognition was not given to how much better hospitals can be, how much more humanly patients can be treated, and how much more kindly we can be.

Ms. Gina Novendstern (Community Health Nurse, Cambridge, Mass.): I want to agree with and expand on what Dr. Prout just said. I, too, work with the losers, with people for whom decisions have been made that they can refuse treatment or die. But no one seems to consider their right to life and the services available to them. Sen. Bertonazzi said that there has not been much public outcry concerning what happens to the patients after a decision has been made to treat them. What about the fact that insurance will not reimburse for terminal care, either at home or in a hospital? Medicare will not reimburse for chronic care of patients who are not receiving the kind of acute care that we are giving them the right to refuse. When we talk about who is going to make decisions and how they are going to be made, we also must explore these issues.

Prof. Annas: That is very insightful. As someone interested in patients' rights for a long time, it has always struck me that the right that is talked about the most is the right to die. And that is really what most patients want the least.

Dr. James H. Gordon (Psychiatrist, Nassau County Medical Center, Great Neck, N.Y.): One of the panel members said that he felt there was an underlying harmony to everything that was going on, even though we may be perturbed about different things; I take some comfort in that. Mr. Chayet suggested that to understand what is going on, lawyers and judges should go see a baby in an incubator. But as a physician, I would say that you should see these babies 100 times and just keep going, because the situation is different all the time. It is a charade to have somebody go in just once. What you see when you are 30 is not what you will see when you are 60. You probably will be much better at handling the situation when you are 60, because you will change as you witness this kind of thing happening over and over. Judges do not want to walk into an intensive care unit, and it is very scary for them to do so. I see this in my practice when I go before judges in mental health information cases. Judges do not have the training and do not want it. They do their best, and they are right most of the time, but you really have to see these cases over and over in order to appreciate your own growth and to help you work with families.

As Prof. Burt said, we have a dilemma, and I hope that everyone who tries to plan procedures realizes that it is going to remain a dilemma. This is living. We live and we die, and ever since death was first recognized, people have been upset about it. That is really all we are talking about here. To have some judge say that we do not have to be upset about it anymore is not going to solve a thing.

A very important article was published some time ago concerning personality types in medical management. There are many different procedures and plans, and sometimes they work. The paternalist is right sometimes, the consumerist is right sometimes, and the advocate or representative is right sometimes. In planning procedures, however, it is very important to realize that different people are involved all the time; there are different answers for different folks, and it is helpful to plan for different kinds of people.

Prof. Annas brushed off the competent person, but I am asked every day whether someone is competent. Maybe another conference should be held on all these competent people, for whom we are happily saying they have no problems because they can make their own decisions. In reality, when someone is sick, everything changes. Competency is a tough area.

Prof. Gadow said we should change to collaborative medicine. My understanding is that medicine has always been collaborative. Doctors do not make these decisions alone, and these decisions are so difficult to make that some people are willing to let judges do it. I don't think families will let that happen.

Concerning the patient representative idea, most patients would not want to talk to a representative; they prefer dealing with physicians. But there are very powerful forces at play here. I think we are trying to forget about the unconscious forces and make them conscious. Remember, whoever talks to the patient also has an unconscious force at work. While you can try to involve people who are more or less removed from the situation, you are never going to get away from unconscious forces and feelings, which will influence what they say.

Prof. Glantz: Responding to Dr. Relman, I want to talk about the pickle we are in now. Asking how we got into this pickle or how we get out is probably the wrong question. The assumption is that the pickle was caused by the *Saikewicz* case, and that is not true. It was there before *Saikewicz*. For example, Prof. Robertson's article on involuntary euthanasia of defective newborns was written before anyone ever heard of *Saikewicz* or *Quinlan*; he pointed out that physicians risk indictment for homicide if they let defective newborns die. Mr. Chayet explained that it is not legally binding for the next of kin to consent to an operation, even though that may be what we have been doing all along; it was not legally binding for us to make decisions about incompetent people even before *Saikewicz*.

Selected Bibliography

Articles and Books

Amundsen, D. W. 1978. The physician's obligation to prolong life: a medical duty without classical roots. *Hastings Cent. Rep.* 8:23–30.

Anderson, R. R. 1969. The physician, the terminal patient and the law. *Lex et Scientia* 6:55–76.

Beauchamp, T. L., and Perlin, S., eds. 1978. *Ethical issues in death and dying.* Englewood Cliffs, N.J.: Prentice-Hall.

Behnke, J. A., and Bok, S., eds. 1975. *The dilemmas of euthanasia.* New York: Doubleday Anchor.

Bok, S. 1976. Personal directions for care at the end of life. *N. Engl. J. Med.* 295:367–369.

Bonnet, J. D., et al. 1975. Symposium issue: euthanasia. *Baylor Law Review* 27:1–108.

Brin, O. G., Jr., et al., eds. 1970. *The dying patient.* New York: Russell Sage Foundation.

Browning, M. H., and Lewis, E. P., eds. 1972. *The dying patient: a nursing perspective.* New York: American Journal of Nursing Co.

Burt, R. A. 1975. Authorizing death for anomalous newborns. In *Genetics and the law*, ed. A. Milunsky and G. Annas. New York: Plenum Press, pp. 435–450.

Byrn, R. M. 1975. Compulsory life saving treatment for the competent adult. *Fordham Law Review* 44:1–36.

Cannon, W. P. 1970. The right to die. *Houston Law Review* 7:654–670.

Cantor, N. L. 1972. A patient's decision to decline life-saving medical treatment: bodily integrity versus the preservation of life. *Rutgers Law Review* 26:228–264.

Conway, D. J. 1974. Medical and legal views of death: confrontation and reconciliation. *St. Louis Univ. Law J.* 19:172–188.

Crane, D. 1975. *The sanctity of social life: physicians' treatment of critically ill patients.* New York: Russell Sage Foundation.

Culliton, B. J. 1975. The Haemmerli affair: is passive euthanasia murder? *Science* 190:1271–1275.

Darling, R. 1977. Parents, physicians, and spina bifida. *Hastings Cent. Rep.* 7:10–13.

Downing, A. B., ed. 1970. *Euthanasia and the right to death.* New York: Humanities Press.

Duff, R. S., and Campbell, A. C. M. 1973. Moral and ethical dilemmas in the special-care nursery. *N. Engl. J. Med.* 289:890–894.

Dyck, A. 1976. The value of life: two contending policies. *Harvard Magazine* (Jan.): 30–36.

Fletcher, G. P. 1967. Prolonging life: some legal considerations. *Washington Law Review* 42:999–1016.

Fletcher, J. C. 1975. Abortion, euthanasia, and care of defective newborns. *N. Engl. J. Med.* 292:75–77.

Fletcher, J. F. 1972. Indicators of humanhood: a tentative profile of man. *Hastings Cent. Rep.* 2:1–4.

Fletcher, J. F. 1974. Four indicators of humanhood—the inquiry matures. *Hastings Cent. Rep.* 4:4–7.

Freeman, J. M. 1972. Is there a right to die—quickly? *J. Pediatr.* 80:904–905. (See also response by R. Cooke, "Whose Suffering?" *ibid.,* 906–908.)

Freeman, J. M. 1973. To treat or not to treat: ethical dilemmas of treating the infant with a myelomeningocele. *Clin. Neurosurg.* 20:134–146.

Gorovitz, S., et al., eds. 1976. *Moral problems in medicine.* Englewood Cliffs, N.J.: Prentice-Hall.

Gruman, G. J. 1973. An historical introduction to ideas about voluntary euthanasia: with a bibliographic survey and guides for inter-disciplinary studies. *Omega* 4:87–138.

Gustafson, J. M. 1973. Mongolism, parental desires, and the right to life. *Perspect. Biol. Med.* 16:529–559.

Hegland, K. F. 1965. Unauthorized rendition of lifesaving medical treatment. *Cal. Law Review* 53:870–877.

Heymann, P. B., and Holtz, S. 1975. The severely defective newborn and the decision process. *Public Policy* 23:381–418.

High, D. M. 1978. Is natural death an illusion? *Hastings Cent. Rep.* 8:37–42.

Humber, J. M., and Almcoer, R. F., eds. 1976. *Biomedical ethics and the law.* New York: Plenum Press.

Hunt, B., and Arras, J., eds. 1977. *Ethical issues in modern medicine.* Palo Alto, Cal.: Mayfield Publishing Co.

Ingelfinger, F. J. 1973. Bedside ethics for the hopeless case. *N. Engl. J. Med.* 289:914–915.

Jonas, H. 1978. The right to die. *Hastings Cent. Rep.* 8:31–36.

Jonsen, A. R., and Garland, M., eds. 1976. *Ethics of newborn intensive care.* San Francisco and Berkeley: University of California School of Medicine and Institute of Government Studies.

Jonsen, A. R., and Lister, G. 1978. Newborn intensive care: the ethical problems. *Hastings Cent. Rep.* 8:15–18.

Jonsen, A. R., et al. 1975. Critical issues in newborn intensive care: a conference report and policy proposal. *Pediatrics* 55:756–764.

Kelsey, B. 1975. Shall these children live? A conversation with Dr. Raymond S. Duff. *Hastings Cent. Rep.* 5:5–8.

Ladd, J., ed. 1979. *Ethical issues relating to life and death.* New York: Oxford University Press.

Langer, W. L. 1974. Infanticide: a historical survey. *History of Childhood Quarterly* 1:353–365.

Levine, C. 1977. Hospital ethics committees: a guarded prognosis. *Hastings Cent. Rep.* 7:25–27.

Lofland, L. H. 1978. *The craft of dying: the modern face of death.* Beverly Hills, Cal.: Sage Publications.

Lorber, J. 1971. Results of treatment of myelomeningocele: an analysis of 524 unselected cases with special reference to possible selection for treatment. *Dev. Med. Child Neurol.* 13:279–303.

Lorber, J. 1974. Selective treatment of myelomeningocele: to treat or not to treat. *Pediatrics* 53:307–308.

McCormick, R. A. 1974. To save or let die: the dilemma of modern medicine. *JAMA* 229:172–176.

McCormick, R. A. 1975. A proposal for "quality of life" criteria for sustaining life. *Hosp. Prog.* (Sept.):76–79.

McCormick, R. A. 1978. The quality of life, the sanctity of life. *Hastings Cent. Rep.* 8:30–36.

McMullin, E., ed. 1978. *Death and decision.* Boulder, Col.: Westview Press.

Montange, C. H. 1974. Informed consent and the dying patient. *Yale Law J.* 83:1632–1634.

Morris, A. A. 1970. Voluntary euthanasia. *Washington Law Review* 45:239–271.

Morris, C. 1969. Resuscitation and the law. *Leg. Med. Annu.* 1:73–90.

O'Connor, A. B., compiler. 1976. *Dying and grief: nursing intervention.* New York: American Journal of Nursing Co.

Optimum care for hopelessly ill patients. A report of the Clinical Care Committee of the Massachusetts General Hospital. 1976. *N. Engl. J. Med.* 295:362–364.

Pius XII. 1957. The Pope speaks, prolongation of life. *Observatore Romano* 4:393–398.

Rabkin, M. T.; Gillerman, G.; and Rice, N. 1976. Orders not to resuscitate. *N. Engl. J. Med.* 295:364–369.

Ramsey, P. 1970. *The patient as person.* New Haven: Yale University Press.

Ramsey, P. 1978. *Ethics at the edges of life.* New Haven: Yale University Press.

Reich, W. 1975. The physician's "duty" to preserve life. *Hastings Cent. Rep.* 5:14–15.

Reid, R. 1977. Spina bifida: the fate of the untreated. *Hastings Cent. Rep.* 7:16–19.

Reiser, S. J.; Dyck, A.; and Curran W., eds. 1977. *Ethics in medicine:*

historical perspectives and contemporary concerns. Cambridge, Mass.: MIT Press.

Robertson, J. A. 1975. Discretionary non-treatment of defective newborns. In *Genetics and the law,* ed. A. Milunsky and G. Annas. New York: Plenum Press, pp. 451–465.

Robertson, J. A. 1975. Involuntary euthanasia of defective newborns: a legal analysis. *Stanford Law Review* 27:213–267.

Schowalter, J. E.; Ferholt, J. B.; and Mann, N. M. 1973. The adolescent patient's decision to die. *Pediatrics* 51:97–103.

Shannon, T. 1977. Caring for the dying patient: what guidance from the guidelines? *Hastings Cent. Rep.* 7:28–30.

Shaw, A. 1973. Dilemmas of "informed consent" in children. *N. Engl. J. Med.* 289:885–890.

Shaw, A. 1977. Defining the quality of life. *Hastings Cent. Rep.* 7:11.

Shaw, A.; Randolph, J. C.; and Manard, B. 1977. Ethical issues in pediatric surgery: a national survey of pediatricians and pediatric surgeons. *Pediatrics* 60 (Suppl.):588–599.

Smith, D. H. 1974. On letting some babies die. *Hastings Cent. Studies* 2 (May):37–46.

Smith, G., and Smith, E. D. 1973. Selection for treatment in spina bifida cystica. *Br. Med. J.* (Oct. 27):189–204.

Steinfels, P., and Veatch, R. M., eds. 1975. *Death inside out.* New York: Harper and Row.

Swinyard, C.A., ed. 1978. *Decision-making and the defective newborn.* Proceedings of the Conference on Spina Bifida and Ethics. Springfield, Ill.: Charles C Thomas.

Thielicke, H. 1970. The doctor as judge of who shall live and who shall die. In *Who shall live?* ed. K. Vaux. Philadelphia: Fortress Press, pp. 147–194.

Todres, I. D.; Krane, D.; Howell, M.; and Shannon, D. 1977. Pediatricians' attitudes affecting decision-making in defective newborns. *Pediatrics* 60:197–201.

Towers, B. 1978. The impact of the California Natural Death Act. *J. Med. Ethics* 4:96–98.

Travis, T. A.; Noyes, R.; and Brightwell, D. R. 1974. The attitudes of physicians toward prolonging life. *Int. J. Psychiatry Med.* 5: 17–26.

Veatch, R. 1976. *Death, dying, and the biological revolution.* New Haven: Yale University Press.

Veatch, R. 1977. Death and dying: the legislative options. *Hastings Cent. Rep.* 7:5–8.

Veatch, R. 1977. Spina bifida: the technical criterion fallacy. *Hastings Cent. Rep.* 7:15–16.

Veatch, R. 1977. Hospital ethics committees: is there a role? *Hastings Cent. Rep.* 7:22–25.

Weber, L. J. 1976. *Who shall live? The dilemma of severely handicapped children and its meaning for other moral questions.* New York: Paulist Press.

Williams, R. H., ed. 1973. *To live and to die.* New York: Springer-Verlag.

Working Party of the Newcastle Regional Hospital Board. 1975. Ethics of selective treatment of spina bifida. *Lancet* 1:85–88.

Legal Decisions

Custody of a Minor
   1978 Mass. Adv. Sh. 2002, 379 N.E.2d 1053 (1978).

In the Matter of Karen Quinlan
   70 N.J. 10, 355 A.2d 647 (1976), cert. denied, 429 U.S. 922 (1976).

In the Matter of Quackenbush
   156 N.J. Super. 282, 383 A.2d 785 (1978).

In the Matter of Shirley Dinnerstein
   1978 Mass. Adv. Sh. 736, 380 N.E.2d 134 (1978).

Lane v. *Candura*
   1978 Mass. App. Adv. Sh. 588, 376 N.E.2d 1232 (1978).

Maine Medical Center v. *Houle*
   Maine Sup. Ct., Civ. Action No. 74–145 (1974).

Satz v. *Perlmutter*
   Fla. App. 326 S.2d 160 (1978).

Shrimp v. *McFall*
   Ct. of Common Pleas, Allegheny Co., Pa. (1978).

State Department of Human Services v. *Northern*
   563 S.W.2d 197 (1978).

Superintendent of Belchertown State School v. *Saikewicz*
   1977 Mass. Adv. Sh. 2461, 370 N.E.2d 417 (1977).

Commentaries on *Quinlan*

Annas, G. J. 1976. *In re Quinlan:* legal comfort for doctors. *Hastings Cent. Rep.* 6:29–31.

Becker, D. W., et al. 1977. The legal aspects of the right to die: before and after the *Quinlan* decision. *Kentucky Law J.* 65:823–879.

Bennett, S. A. 1976. In the shadow of Karen Quinlan. *Trial* 12:36–41.

Berger, P. F., and Berger, C. A. 1975. Death on demand: the complexity of the *Quinlan* case overwhelms traditional thinking. *Commonweal* CII:585–589.

Branson, R., and Casebeer, K. 1976. The *Quinlan* decision: obscuring the role of the physician. *Hastings Cent. Rep.* 6:8–11.

Capron, A. M. 1976. The *Quinlan* decision: shifting the burden of decision making. *Hastings Cent. Rep.* 6:17–19.

Coburn, D. R. 1977. *In re Quinlan* (NJ) 355 A.2d 647: a practical overview. *Arkansas Law Review* 31:59–74.

Connery, J. R. 1976. The *Quinlan* case. *Linacre Quarterly* 43:25–28.

Doty, R. 1976. Constitutional law—no constitutional basis exists to permit a parent to assert for his adult child a right to die. *Texas Tech. Law Review* 7:716–723.

Hastings Center Report. 1976. Commentaries on the *Quinlan* case. 6:8–19.

Healey, J. M., Jr. 1976. The *Quinlan* case and the mass media. *Am. J. Public Health* 66:295–296.

Hyland, W. F., and Balme, D. S. 1976. *In re Quinlan* [(NJ) 355 A.2d 647]: a synthesis of law and medical technology. *Rutgers Camden Law J.* 8:37–64.

In the matter of Karen Quinlan: the complete legal briefs, court proceedings and decision in the Superior Court of New Jersey, Vol. I, 1975; Vol. II, 1976. Arlington, Va.: University Publications of America.

In re Quinlan: a symposium. 1977. *Rutgers Law Review* 30:243–328.

In re Quinlan [(NJ) 355 A.2d 647]: one court's answer to the problem of death with dignity. 1977. *Washington and Lee Law Review* 34:285–308.

Kennedy, I. McC. 1976. The Karen Quinlan case: problems and proposals. *J. Med. Ethics* 2:3–7.

Levine, M. D. 1976. The *Quinlan* decision: disconnection: the clinician's view. *Hastings Cent. Rep.* 6:11–12.

McCormick, R. A. 1976. The moral right to privacy: commentary on the *Quinlan* decision. *Hosp. Prog.* 57:38–42.

Oden, T. C. 1976. The *Quinlan* decision: beyond an ethic of immediate sympathy. *Hastings Cent. Rep.* 6:12–14.

Ramsey, P. 1976. The *Quinlan* decision: prolonged dying: not medically indicated. *Hastings Cent. Rep.* 6:14–17.

Ramsey, P. 1978. *Ethics at the edges of life.* New Haven: Yale University Press, ch. 7.

Rome, H. P. 1976. More about Karen Ann Quinlan. *Psychiatric Annals* 6:97–105.

Shannon, T. A. 1975. A triumph of technology: the technological imperative of the *Quinlan* case. *Commonweal* CII:589–590.

Smith, W. F. 1976. *In re Quinlan* [(NJ) 355 A.2d 647]: defining the basis for terminating life support under right of privacy. *Tulsa Law Review* 12:150–167.

Vaux, K. L. 1976. Beyond this place: spiritual and ethical issues in the *Quinlan* case. *Christian Century* (Jan. 21):43–47.

Who should decide? The case of Karen Quinlan. 1976. *Christianity and Crisis* 35:322–331.

Commentaries on *Saikewicz*

Annas, G. 1978. After *Saikewicz:* no fault death. *Hastings Cent. Rep.* 8:16–18.

Annas, G. 1978. The incompetent's right to die: the case of Joseph Saikewicz. *Hastings Cent. Rep.* 8:21–23.

Annas, G. 1979. Reconciling *Quinlan* and *Saikewicz:* decision making for the terminally ill incompetent. *Am. J. Law Med.* 4:367–396. (See additional references therein to *Quinlan, Saikewicz,* and *Dinnerstein.*)

Baron, C. 1978. Assuring "detached but passionate investigation and decision": the role of guardians-ad-litem in *Saikewicz*-type cases. *Am. J. Law Med.* 4:111–130.

Curran, W. J. 1978. The *Saikewicz* decision. *N. Engl. J. Med.* 298:499–500. (See also letters to the editor, *ibid.* 298:1208–1209.)

The decision to die—who makes it? (editorial). 1978. *Mass. Lawyers Weekly* 6:596.

Dumanoski, D. 1978. In the matter of life and death. *The Boston Phoenix*, 23 May, p. 6ff.

Glantz, L., and Swazey, J. 1979. Decisions not to treat: the *Saikewicz* case and its aftermath. *Forum on Medicine* 2:22–32.

McCormick, R. A., and Hellegers, A. E., 1978. The specter of Joseph Saikewicz: mental incompetence and the law. *America* (Apr.): 257–260.

Ramsey, P. 1978. *Ethics at the edges of life.* New Haven: Yale University Press, ch. 8.

Relman, A. S. 1978. The *Saikewicz* decision: judges as physicians. *N. Engl. J. Med.* 298:508–509.

Bibliographic Sources

Bibliography of society, ethics and life sciences. Annual. Hastings-on-Hudson, N.Y.: Institute of Society, Ethics, and the Life Sciences.

Bioethicsline. National Library of Medicine's computerized online bibliographic data base. Inquire at medical school libraries or contact BIOETHICSLINE, Center for Bioethics, Kennedy Institute, Georgetown University, Washington, D.C. 20057.

Clouser, D. K., and Zucker, A. 1974. *Abortion and euthanasia: an annotated bibliography.* Philadelphia: Society for Health and Human Values.

Fulton, R., et al., compilers. 1977. *Death, grief, and bereavement: a bibliography, 1845–1975.* New York: Arno Press.

Goldstein, D. M. 1973. *A bibliography of bibliographies in bioethics.* Washington, D.C.: Georgetown University.

Kutscher, M. L., et al. 1975. *A comprehensive bibliography of the thanatology literature.* New York: Mss Information Co.

Newsletter on Science, Technology and Human Values. Cambridge, Mass.: Harvard Program on Science, Technology and Public Policy (published quarterly).

Nick, W. V. 1970. *Index of legal medicine, 1940–1970: an annotated bibliography.* Columbus, Ohio: Legal Medicine Press (updated by pamphlet supplements).

Sell, I. 1977. *Death and dying: an annotated bibliography.* New York: The Tiresias Press.

Walters, L., ed. *Bibliography of bioethics.* Detroit, Mich.: Gale Research Co. (published annually).